Blue **Print**

Advice, Adventures, and Cougar Tales

———&———

[handwritten inscription:] ale / e said TOMORROW / STERDAY! Make it / appen TODAY!! ♡ Ava

Blue **Print**

Advice, Adventures, and Cougar Tales

———🖇———

AVA G. BLACK
MISSION POSSIBLE PRESS, USA
Creating Legacies through Absolute Good Works
Aspiration Publishing Series

Blue Print
Advice, Adventures and Cougar Tales
Copyright © 2015 Ava G. Black AvaGBlack.wordpress.com

Aspiration Publishing: Solutions for Life's Problems
For those who have a strong desire to achieve something high
or great.

MISSION POSSIBLE PRESS
P.O. Box 8039
St. Louis, MO 63156
Publisher@AbsoluteGood.com

ISBN: 978-0-9861818-1-8
Printed in the United States of America

Contents

———— 🖇 ————

Introduction
Ahhhh... Finally Exhaling!

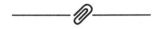

Hello and welcome to the world of Ms. Ava G. Black. It's been a LONG time coming and it's finally here. I have dreamed of a book which allows me to share what I have learned over the years. To say what's on my mind, and likely in the minds and hearts of many women just like me. While we're each unique with our own special way of navigating life, men and women are really not all that different from one another. I believe my sentiments express what women *should be* thinking and feeling. Here, I get to express those thoughts without the stigma of being politically or sexually incorrect.

The following words will take on different meanings for different people depending on where you might be in your life journey. Whatever it means to you is what it's *supposed* to mean. I simply hope I can be a worthy guide and host for your inner most thoughts. Those thoughts you'd *never* dream of sharing with anyone because you thought they were just too much or too crazy. They aren't.

Whether we agree or disagree, it can be neither right nor wrong. It's just me... and just you. NOTHING is off limits. Language is not an issue. And I share myself in the same way I would when talking to close friends - with great respect, limited judgment (nobody's perfect), and no name calling unless referring to self.

I've come to a place in my life where I have learned some hard yet valuable lessons and feel the need to share. That's what I would have wanted from a wiser more experienced woman. Maybe the opportunity never presented itself. Maybe she didn't feel comfortable sharing. Or maybe, just maybe, she really didn't have a clue either.

It's why I want to share with everyone. Not just my close friends and intellectual equals, but with the younger twenty something's as well. Hopefully, this information will effectively change the way you see sex and relationship issues. If nothing else, I want women to understand one thing - the way a man acts in a relationship is rarely, IF EVER, personal. It's just who they are and how they think. But the playing field can be leveled...and this can be the beginning of that understanding.

For the fellas, pay attention. I make no apologies for the lessons I've learned and share. This is the end of success with random bullshit. Be prepared to step it up, or get out of the way of the man who will. Feel free to call me out on anything should you feel the need. I can be reached anonymously at AvaGBlack. wordpress.com.

Man or woman – Happy Reading! I don't know about you but I LOOOOVE talking about, thinking about, and actually having sex! My mind is forever open, and so is the door to my sexual soul!!

Buckle up and enjoy the ride!
Ava G.

Preface
The Roar of a Woman

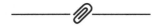

There are a few things you should know before you settle into my theories on life, love, sex, and relationships.

First, I've been married twice and divorced twice, both times for love (idiot moves). My first husband was a nice enough guy. We never really fought and had great sex... just not often enough. That got old after a while and I bitched about it all the time. My constant complaining about not getting enough sex, and his refusal to give in to me as often as I would have liked, led to problems in and out of the bedroom. Even in my mid-twenties I was a big fan of sex. That's crazy because I barely even knew what I was doing, and I was still faking orgasms (a crime against humanity). Long story short - he turned out to be gay. He has never come out and likely never will. However, trust me – he is. Needless to say, it didn't work out. No big fights, no big scenes, we just went our separate ways, no hard feelings. Every girlfriend he had after we divorced reached out to ask me if we ever had sex problems and if he was gay. I never revealed or dished. But I should have known something was up when the pastor asked him the same thing during a counseling session. His frat brothers and best friends had a sit down intervention with him years later assuring him they didn't care and would still be there for him. But he has still refused to be himself.

My second husband has been far more difficult to shake. Five years post-divorce and I can't remember three days when he hasn't sent me some kind of hate email or text. It has taken a moment, but I have learned to ignore him and I am better for it. We were friends for almost fifteen years before a weak moment turned into a marriage which pretty much ruined me. Regardless, I have learned who I am and grown from both experiences in every way possible, and I survived.

Second, I don't like labels. Never have. The idea that a person can be summed up in a word just makes no sense to me. Things are never that easy. There are always exceptions to every rule, and lots of gray areas. Not to mention almost every word in the English language can mean something different to every person. I may refer to myself in terms of what I may be feeling for the moment, but it is rarely an acceptance of an overall characteristic of myself defined by society. 'Cougar' is a good example.

In case you are not familiar: **Cougar** – [**koo**-ger]; NOUN. An attractive woman her late 30's – early 40's or older, who generally looks much younger than she should and is 'on the hunt' to date younger men; age gap is usually a minimum of at least ten years. I honestly had never heard the term until a few years ago, right after turning forty.

I had a kick-ass birthday party with a running theme of 'Thirty-Is-The-New-Forty' (it continues). Well into the night, following many, many drinks, and top shelf tequila shots, while laying on top of the pool table, my cousin approached to see if I was ok, and needed or wanted anything. I said, "Yes! A cute guy to dance with!" Seconds later she poked me to get up. I rose to see a beeee-you-tee-ful man in front of me. I looked at him. I looked at her. I squealed, "That's for me cuz!?!"

He set the standard from then to current day. A month later we were booked in a hotel room for the weekend. We didn't even leave for food. It was non-stop amazing for three days! Non-stop amazing. He ruined me for age appropriate men. It was the first time *in my life*, I didn't have to wait. No recovery time. *No recovery time!* I felt like I was in a damn dream. There have been countless weekends since then, each better than the last. Who would **ever** willingly give that up?! Not your girl Ava!!!

So, while cougar is probably one of my least favorite society appointed titles, I've come to love and embrace it. Call me whatever you want if it means unlimited orgasms with a sexy man who only wants to please ME.

Third - I don't date. I have no interest in being anyone's girlfriend or wife, so why bother? I have my favorites, but there is always an open spot on Ava's roster. Plus, we're talking about *attracting* younger men. Dating them is a complete waste of time. I've dated a few and it always ends badly for them, and I always feel guilty about it. They think they're in love because the sex is good. Marriage proposals follow. Not cool. So now I don't let that happen. I don't date. If the chemistry is there, I go with it. If not, I don't. It's my choice and I am brutal in making it these days. I find myself wishing some of them would not feel the need to converse. *Just shut up and stay in your lane please*, is what I want them to do.

Men are definitely safe from 'all things emotional' with me. The only thing that gets me emotional is multiple orgasms. That ish can make me cry. I am in my sexual prime, and if I have learned nothing over the past fifteen years or so, it's how to have amazing sex which is completely detached from anything other than the physical. Men over forty just piss me off in the bedroom. Judge me if you must but I make no apologies for either.

I would suggest you kick back, grab a glass of wine, and chill. Talking about sex is almost as much fun as having it. I'd love your feedback and welcome you to share your thoughts confidentially. It is my hope the experiences and advice I share in the next few pages will inspire conversations between friends, and empower women who are learning to appreciate themselves, say what they feel, and care less about what other people think or want to hear.

Chapter 1
Of Course Size Matters!

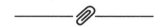

Dear Ava,

I have one question. Does size really matter? I hope you say no because I almost want to be told to stop being petty. I'm 28 and I've been with my boyfriend for 8 months. The sex is good, but I know it can be better. He is much smaller than what I am used to and would like. It feels fine, I guess, but I want better than fine. I have been missing my ex-boyfriend lately. The thing is, I don't want him back I just miss how it felt when he was inside me. No matter what was going on between us, the sex was always good and I found it very hard to say no even when I was really pissed at him. I don't want to break up with my current boyfriend and I don't want to get back with my ex. But, not returning his calls is getting more and more difficult. Does size really matter in the long run? Help me understand what I can do to get past this petty issue when I have a great guy.

Signed,
'My Girl' is Unhappy

Blue **Print**

Well Unhappy,   ✍

I wish I could tell you what you want to hear. I wish I could tell you that size doesn't matter and you are being petty. I wish I could tell you to stop tripping and get over yourself... but I just can't lie to you girl. Size definitely matters! If it didn't, you wouldn't be feeling this way! It's not your fault you've been 'exposed' to some big D. I'm actually kinda jealous! I was over 30 when I got my first taste of 'the good life.' Already once married and divorced, it scared me to think I could have gone the rest of my life without any big D. had I stayed married. Pheeeww - I really dodged a bullet with that!

I am going to suggest a few things. None of them have anything to do with love or emotion with regard to your relationship. Not only because I think it's completely unrelated, but because I don't think you should have to sacrifice something you want, to be happy loving someone else. You have to love yourself first.

That's something women are always happy to do...take the back-burner. Stop that! We matter! What you want matters! If you've had big D, and you like big D, then get BIG D and be happy! That doesn't mean I think you should go back to your ex. He's an ex for a reason so remember that. But exercise your options!

First - throw honesty out the window. I haven't met a man yet who could handle hearing the truth about his beloved package. No matter how hard you try to find the words, there is no delicate way to say, 'You have a small dick and it ain't working for me.' Plus, he won't believe you because NO woman has ever said that to him before, and he believes every woman he's ever touched has orgasmed like crazy. That's our fault for always faking them.

Second - toys. Toys might be able to save you. You have to go about it in a way that screams, 'I'm ready to show you my inner freak,' versus 'We need help and this is my last ditch effort before cheating on or dropping you.' Since you care about him, make it easy for him. Be prepared to suffer through at least a few more weeks of being dissatisfied. Creatively bring up the subject of toys, and then reluctantly agree to a late night trip to an adult store. He'll love taking you there because every man secretly wants a whore in the bedroom, and lady in the streets. Fortunately, almost all of us can be both if we want to. Buy a few minor 'upgrades' (i.e. edible lotions, etc) and let things progress from there. It will take some time but eventually you can grab a decent vibrator and it might work for you. If not, maybe you'll see one that could work for you when he's not around, and you can go back and get it for yourself.

Third - be prepared to bounce. This is a temporary fix. This man will never be able to give you what you want in the long run. He will never amount to your ex. Relationships are tough and require work and dedication. At some point, the little d will take its toll on you. If you stay with him and try to build a life, when things get tough you will cheat to at least get what you want physically. Just remember, you deserve to be HAPPY and I believe everyone's idea of their total package is out there. You need to figure out what's in yours.

It's all about you,

Ava

***

I see absolutely no point in beating around the bush, so to speak. Does size really matter? Some would say no. They would be lying. Size does matter in just about everything. As a society overall we all want everything bigger, SUPER sized! Wouldn't it be great if it were that easy to get the perfect male sex organ?

Imagine meeting someone, getting to know him, and really liking him. The customary and acceptable number of dates has been fulfilled and as you draw nearer to "the big reveal" you are filled with anticipation, excitement, and angst. Your prayers are filled with requests of massive rewards. I mean, ... *he's almost perfect in every other way so please, please, please let his manhood be representative of his manhood...* You're in the moment. There is no lack of passion. You're ravenous for each other. Tops are off, your hands slide down his six pack, or slight poof of a belly, and you slowly unzip his jeans. Your hand is stretched for the full palm grab and as you make the connection, you chest deflates. *Where is it?* You force your hand from patting around in there like you lost something important. Inside you're crying. Passion has left the room, the moment, and the relationship. Now you want to place an order, "Larger penis please!"

If you have not experienced a moment like this one, trust me... you will. That night will continue like many others before it. He is completely unaware of the monumental shift he just created in your world. You can't and don't want to deal with it right now, or ever, so you just continue and go with the very slow, tear jerking flow. He thinks you are moved to tears by emotion and just being close to him. He is not completely wrong. The source of the emotion is where you differ. The highlight? You know the oral will likely be life changing. It has to be right? There are certain equations which never fail. 'Little Penis = Extended Foreplay + Amazing Oral' almost every time. It just is what it is. But how long is that going to be enough?

I have often wondered, *Is it a subconscious reality for the man with a smaller dick to BE nice BECAUSE he has no dick, or is it a conscious choice?* At what point in his sexual travels does he realize he MUST master cunnilingus? When does it become apparent to him he needs to be a good listener, an excellent communicator, and get to know the va-j better than his more ample and therefore more desirable counterparts?

Regardless of the formula, there isn't a woman alive who hasn't convinced herself, at some point in her life, she can deal with it, myself included. We ask ourselves, *How important is sex anyway?* In the *long run* isn't it all about compatibility and companionship? Those self-inflicted mind games might work for a minute. But unless you're willing to settle for toys and let go of hope his penis will actually *get* bigger, you will never be able to sustain it. Foreplay is no substitute for a nice finish. Unless you're a closet lesbian, you're gonna need the real deal penis at the end of every session and I'm guessing a strap on for your man is not an option. Speaking of strap ons, even lesbians like big D! Small dick pleases no one.

Is it fair that most often Asshole Man = Huge Penis + Game Player? No. But again I have to ask myself, is it a subconscious reality for the man with the larger penis to be an ass *because* he has what every woman wants and cannot resist? Why else would a woman go back time and time again to the same jerk of a man who has no idea what it means to *be* a spouse or a keeper of hearts? Just like a man can be whipped, oh how we woman can succumb to the D!

We want to believe the little-dick nice guy can satisfy us in other ways. After all, orgasms are nice and of course it's the ultimate goal. When done well, most women easily reach it via oral stimulation (yes easily... when done *well*). It stands to reason if this is a guaranteed way to orgasm, what difference does the size of his penis matter if he is a cunnilingus master? However, the only thing a woman wants more than a good oral orgasm is a nice, fat dick to follow it up. Sadly, at some point we will be forced to settle for what he has, or look outside of the relationship for sexual satisfaction. While these may not be the most politically correct or morally acceptable solutions, they are options none the less, until there's some way to place your very own customized order.

Chapter 2
Young Body, Old D!

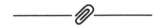

Dear Ava, ✍

As a women in my sexual prime (42), how can I be sexually satisfied without resorting to young guns? My boyfriend is 45 and he cannot keep up! He is good for 30 or 40 minutes tops, on a good day. It's usually a lot shorter. Physically he looks great. He's in good shape, has a wonderful piece, and I can barely keep my hands off him. But he begs for too much time to recover. I find myself getting angry with him lately because he conks out and I am left mad and frustrated even after having a decent orgasm. My sex drive is on overload. How can I maintain my great relationship with him, and still be satisfied sexually? I'm struggling to stay faithful. Can you help?

Signed,
Falling Short

Oh Falling Short,   ✍

I have wondered the same thing. First – talk to him. He won't listen or believe you because he thinks he is 'putting it down' (and maybe he is). But still let him know how you feel. He probably wants to give you all that you want... he just can't! He's not twenty-five anymore! Suggest cardio for stamina and weight lifting for lifting your weight (because we all love to be properly tossed). And after all of that just know... none of it will help or matter!

This is why I firmly believe women in their forties are sexual perfection for a man in his prime at twenty-one to thirty. All the running, hiking, climbing, and weight lifting in the world will change nothing below the waist for your man. His manhood will always scream "I'm forty-two and this woman is trying to kill me!"

Brace yourself - my suggestion is to nurture your age appropriate relationship fully, and get your cougar on in your spare time. Yes, I just encouraged you to seek sexual satisfaction elsewhere! Let's face it, he will never be able to keep up with you at his age. You have to know your prime will not last forever, just look at how long it took to get here! What do you think our boyfriends did during their prime?

As a woman, a grown azzz woman, you know how to be discreet and not get caught out there. Go get yours and stop falling short girl!

Never Settle,

Ava

It's just natural that every woman feels this way at one time or another. Scientifically, women don't truly hit their stride until much later than men. We are never on the same sexual clock. When we are feeling the emotional connections in high school and college, men are looking for the next opportunity to be inside of any *body*. When we finally understand how it's even possible to have sex without being in love or having some kind of emotional connection, many of us are married with kids and forced to fight the biological urges to seek outside assistance. Well, some of us fight them.

Thankfully, my clock didn't 'kick-in' until after I was done being married. Knowing what I know now, I can't say I would have been able to ward off a twenty-five year old sexual tiger just as I was finally beginning to understand the whole, 'Babe-it-didn't-mean-anything-it-was-just-sex' story. A woman in her forties will feel this way eventually. Where the emotional used to control, the physical now trumps. I knew this to be true when, at forty-two, I reconnected with my first boyfriend.

We had not been together since we were sixteen, but oh does the heart remember. I loved this man and 'muscle memory' was in full swing. He was my first kiss, my first love, my first everything. When we met up face-to-face the stars must have been aligned. Our feelings reemerged for one another and were instantaneously, a very big deal. It certainly didn't hurt that he had a beautiful, crazy, chiseled body. It's just ridiculous. A body perfectly made for eyeing and fanaticizing. Constructed like he was drawn on a piece of paper and had just leapt off the page. I don't intimidate easily but his body was just *crazy.* He looks really good. Still.

After months of talking, and basically falling in some kind of love again, we hooked up. Music on, lights off, he walked into hotel the room, flicked on the light, and picked up the TV remote. Three hours later, I climbed on top of him because I was tired of waiting. I can watch TV at home. The sex was good and I was immediately ready to go again. And then a whiny little girl seemed to appear in our room.

She looked like a man, sounded like a man, but the words were all *cry baby whining*. When I reached for him he asked what I was doing. He acted as if he was just found in the Sahara after days of crawling for shade. "I need water, cold water, and a little time, for real. I need some rest and down time." Excuse me WHAT?! I was annoyed but what can you do?

I waited fifteen minutes and the whiny girl was back in our room, "What are you doing? I don't have anything else. I'm seriously going to need some time. Give me thirty more minutes." I'm pretty sure he started snoring *while* he was talking. I left him alone for about three hours. Two hours after that he reluctantly 'hooked me up.' I'm pretty sure it was out of sympathy. He was truly done afterwards. "I can't recover that quick girl. Damn! I need *complete* down time." So, I left him alone for another four hours. When I woke him up for more he was irate. He told me he didn't know what was wrong with me, but he was damn proud of himself because he hadn't performed that way in twenty years!

This is what being with men in their twenties has done to me.

His body was banging and I didn't understand how he could look so good and be so fit, yet not be able to continue to have sex. He explained, "I have stamina to run but that doesn't have anything to do with the stamina of my D. My D is forty-two and my D cannot be lied to." I wanted more but it was an 'aha moment.' He literally took my hand off his D and pushed it away. Six hours between sessions and he had nothing left. I finally understood.

A forty-two year old man being in good physical shape helps with stamina and sex appeal, but it has *nothing to* do with the stamina of his dick. Did you get that?! Let me say that one more time because understanding it changed my life: A man can be in the best physical shape of his life (six pack, and all), but his forty plus year old 'partna from down under' will NOT reflect it! He will not be able to keep up with a woman in her prime! The reality that men date women in their twenties *not only* because they look good, but because they demand little! Bang, bang, bang away!

That weekend I learned a lot. He showed me that the forty-two year old D couldn't do me up the way I was used to being done up by twenty something D. All that talk about love and getting back together was O-VER. I was no longer even remotely interested in being with him anymore. Since he couldn't give me any the next day either, I ended up checking out of the hotel two days early and taking my ass back to what I could count on. Sex once a day in hotel room is unacceptable. The physical has trumped the emotional ever since.

After the trip he seemed angry. Being angry was mutual, for different reasons. We were both over each other. We discussed having a do over. He thinks he's ready. I'm good. By his own logic, he will *never* be ready. He calls me 'The Destroyer' claiming I am ruining the young guns for other women. I not-so-secretly hope that's true.

Chapter 3
Cougars Love Young Guns!

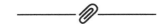

Dear Ava,

I want to be a cougar! Where do I sign up? I'm 37 and just can't seem to find a younger man to have fun with. I've been to clubs and parties with my younger girlfriends and still nothing! It's so frustrating because I really want this! I meet plenty of men but they are all my age or older and I don't want to be bothered. What do I have to do to be like you and 'pull the young ones?'

Signed,
Teacher By Nature

Teacher, Teacher, Teacher.

I really can't tell you what you have to do to "pull the young ones." They just come to me. It's who I meet when I'm out. I don't really club much, maybe twice in the last two years? But that doesn't matter, men love sexy women. If you take care of yourself, and feel like a sexy, exciting, and beautiful women who carries herself as such... they will come.

My entry into the realm wasn't purposeful. It just happened because I was constantly being approached by younger men who had no idea I was an older woman. Most guessed me at close to their own age, or slightly younger. Being a cougar isn't something you need to go out and hunt to be (ironically). It just happens. It seems to me you have a bigger problem...

You want to be with a younger man more than you want to be with a man! You meet "plenty of men" but you don't want to be bothered? Girl, please! If you are shaking them off like that, no wonder the young ones are afraid to approach! Think about it. They are young. Shy. Nervous. They are just learning how this game works and if anyone is interested in you, watching you swat men off like flies is not going to be good for their young, fragile egos. Yes, it's harsh, but it's true.

Just remember, someone is always watching. You have to be approachable. You don't need to give your number to every man that asks, but you need to be nice and refuse it with a smile. I can't even count how many men have approached me to rescue me from someone I obviously was not interested in. A smile will get you a long way, especially when it can be seen from across the room.

Plus, I have nothing against any man. While we all have our preferences, I'm attracted to men, not a number. If he's sexy, smart, and makes me laugh, why would I walk away from that? The problem I generally find with 'older men' is their inability to keep up in the bedroom. If that's all you're looking for, stop waiting for who you want to approach you and make the first move. If all you want is sex, then saying the first hello is the easy part!

Enjoy the ride missy!
Ava

***

It was at my fortieth birthday party which started all of this for me. It was completely by accident and an extension of my desire *not* to be forty! I had a private room in one of the hottest 'young' clubs in the area. My friends were excited to get the invitation because they'd heard about this club, but of course would have never gone to be with such young people. In fact, one of my closest girlfriends couldn't make it but I ran into her daughter at the club! That was creepy! I was there when this child was born and now she was running up to me in a club screaming, "Auntie, Auntie!" I looked at her like she'd snuck in with fake ID when actually, I was the one who probably shouldn't have been there!

But there I was, in a room filled with 'all things thirty!' Around 4am when my cousins said it was time to go, my sexy 'gifted' dance partner grabbed me around the waist and bent down to ask me for my number. I turned around, hugged him and told him he was too young for me but thanks for the fun night. He laughed and insisted he wasn't *that* young. I guessed him at twenty-five and hit it dead on. He looked confused, and leaned back to peek into my room, observing all the thirty something's in there. Looking back at me he very nonchalantly said, "Babe, that's only 5 years."

Now I was confused. Did this man *really* think I was turning thirty? I laughed out loud and hard. Wondering what I thought was so funny, he started telling me age was just a number and blah, blah, blah. I heard nothing after a while. *Did this man REALLY think I was turning thirty!?!* Were my only thoughts. I just couldn't wrap my head around it.

I finally confessed, leaning up and whispering my real age into his ear. He was shocked. He stepped back and looked me up and down. It felt good, how he looked at me. "I don't believe you, but I also don't care," he said. He asked me to repeat it twice more. That also felt good. He stepped back again and said it was impossible. I must have completely blacked out for a moment. Completely uninhibited by logic or decency, I stood on my toes, pulled him close, and was kissing him full on in seconds. Was that an improper thank you?

Kissing him felt goooood. He was young and sexy, and

thought I was too! What could be more exciting than that?! I was loving my forties! I don't even remember giving him my number, but he called me a day or so later and I was glad! We'd spend hours on the phone and it quickly became all about touching and sex. I mean, what else were we going to talk about? He was super excited to be with an older woman, and I was over-the-moon that I was starting my forties off feeling a twenty-five year old again! There were five states between us so we quickly began planning for a weekend to meet in the middle.

Before I knew it, I was deplaning and looking forward to twenty-five! Wooo hooooo! We booked an extended stay hotel with a full kitchen, living room, etc. I ran to the market and grabbed a few staples. Food for eating, food for fun, and the ingredients for his favorite drink. I arrived about two hours before him and 'set up' the room.

Setting up the room was especially fun. Over the years I had gone to great lengths in various relationships to be romantic, wear lingerie, and set the mood. Reactions were varied. Everything from straight laughter, to lights being flicked on, to "cute babe" types of comments followed by instructions to take it off. I took this opportunity to really enjoy myself and go all out with my own fantasies. After all, I knew he had never experienced a 'real' woman and not only did I want to make it special and memorable, I wanted to blow his mind the way he imagined a forty year old woman could.

First thing I did was place all my tea light candles strategically around the room. I had about four in the living area, one in the kitchen, and one in the bathroom. No need for lights. One of my candles was special; an especially fragrant soy candle which melted down to massage oil instead of wax. It came with a little spoon for dipping and drizzling. I couldn't wait to try that out. I lit it about an hour before his arrival to make sure the room would smell delish when he walked in. I pulled the blankets down off the bed and sprayed the sheets with a mist of body spray which matched the scent of the candle, and made it up again. Speakers and music were set, with a playlist of sexy ballads on random for the next ten hours. The rest of 'set-up' involved me. My body. My hair. My attitude.

Preparing for sex at forty is a lot more involved than stripping down for the quick 'bang bang' sessions of my twenties. Knowing he was used to the visual of twenty year olds was added pressure. Two kids in, a fresh mani-pedi, brows, bikini wax (Brazilians are for crazy people), and shopping for lingerie, and new bra and panty sets days prior, just didn't seem enough. I did a quick fashion show to decide which to start with and chose red. Freshly showered and oiled up, I dabbed extra doses of my chosen scent and applied it to all the necessary places: Neck, behind the ears, inside biceps, inner thigh, lower back, top-o-the-crack, and behind the knees.

When I got the text that he'd landed and was on his way, I primped my hair, brushed my teeth, climbed into my sexy, vibrant, red number with matching panties, slipped on my sexiest black patent heels, threw on the jeweled candy necklace that looked like rhinestones, and applied a sexy edible chocolate garter just below the bottom of my outfit. I grabbed the shaker and martini glasses I'd brought from home and quickly mixed our martinis and poured. Drapes pulled (it was 2pm), candles lit, lights out, and I was leaning against the door waiting for the knock. When he lightly tapped the door, I took a deep breath, sucked everything in, fluffed the hair, and cracked the door just enough for him to enter.

He walked into our candlelit room, saw the drinks on the kitchen counter, and turned around to see me closing the door and stepping towards him. His jaw dropped, then his bag, and kissing commenced. After we finished an amazingly sensual kiss, his "Hey Baby," was the beginning of an amazing three days. Fourteen condoms. Yes, fourteen!!! At least four fulfilled fantasies were crossed off my sexual bucket list. Of course, a few were pulled off prematurely, but for damn good reason. His energy level was crazy. *I* even experienced a few firsts. The most astonishing: He kept going after cumming, and came again in another twenty minutes, then over and over and over again!! Who the hell needs sleep? I'll sleep when I'm dead... which is around the same time I'd be willing to give all that up! Who the hell would ever let that go? I was in damn heaven!

The past six years have been a never-ending treasure trove of sensationally fulfilled fantasies for both of us, a complete win-win. I joke every now and then that he's gotten to be too old for me now that he's thirty. I think he took me seriously for a minute and seemed to kick himself into overdrive. Motivation is a good thing. And trust, Ava ain't going *anywhere* Babe. Best birthday gift I've ever gotten. The gift that *truly* keeps on giving! Thanks again cuz!

Chapter 4
The Cougar Code

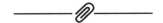

Dear Ava, ✍

I have been a cougar since before it was cool to be one. I consider myself a pioneer; one who has paved the way. It's been fun. I've dated men twenty years my junior, and when we're out, we rarely get a second look. I look DAMN good! My problem is I'm in love with one and we want to marry. Is it crazy to think we could make it even though he's younger than my oldest child?

Signed,
I Wanna Keep Him

Ummm, yeah, Wanna! ✍

It is crazy! I hate to break it to you at this late stage of your weak ass game, but you are no cougar! You've broken so many rules and crossed so many lines I don't even know where to start. His being younger than your oldest child is the least of it.

*I guess you didn't get the memo: Cougars don't date!
Dating is for people who want to get to know each
other and figure out where things could lead. Cougars
know it leads nowhere except the bedroom! Dating is
for grown ups!!*

*Cougar's have. Cougars do. Cougars enjoy. Cougars
indulge. Cougars do not date! Where exactly do you
think the road you've paved leads? You may look
amazing and BE amazing, but you are lacking in good
dayum sense.*

*Cougars by definition are non-committal. We are not
looking to settle down, start a family, or build a life!
Sounds like you've already done that and the plan failed!
Thankfully we still look good enough to have some fun
to make up for it! Your actions are unacceptable.*

*Out? Out?!! I can't think of one good reason why
anyone would ever be out with a younger man except
the moment you meet, and maybe one other time.
What the hell for? You meet. You flirt. There's sexual
attraction and chemistry. You exchange numbers. He
calls. You talk and flirt some more. Conversations
eventually become sexual, intentions are revealed, and
taaaaa-daaaa... plans are made!*

*It's unfair for you to entertain his declaration of love
and you certainly shouldn't be reciprocating it. He
should be dating, but not dating you! He needs to
have the opportunity to meet GIRLS! Young guns are
for great sex with no strings or drama. I'm not saying
you shouldn't expect him to fall for you, as good sex
tends to impair judgment. But have some decency*

and recognize it as such. Cougars don't get sprung, we spring. I don't know what to call what you have been doing but unless you are sixty, and he is forty something, back away slowly and keep it moving!

Obey the rules!

Ava

***

Being a cougar is the biggest and most rewarding side effect to looking younger. I always know when a man is younger than me. Not only by their looks, but once they start talking you can tell. They're nervous and the conversation can be weak. It's kind of cute that they have no idea what they are walking into.

Let's face it, when a man walks towards a woman in any situation to start a conversation, we have already decided if we'd prefer he keep walking. Cougar or not, a woman knows within minutes, five at the most, whether or not she wants a man. At least I do. Sex appeal is sex appeal. It's what follows our realization that becomes the biggest issue. This is where most men either ruin that sexy vibe, or solidify it. Tall, attractive, sexy, funny - all required. The quicker you can relay this with the least amount of stupid as possible = SCORE!

By the way fellas - less really is more. Quiet is so much sexier than stupid. If you only knew just how often you've talked yourself out of some good pussy, you'd be crying real tears right now. For goodness sake, just shut the hell up! That's first-class advice for every man, no matter his age, but especially the older variety, thirty-two and up. Young ones can get a pass because even if they are complete idiots they are still learning and can make up for it in the bedroom, so who cares. Stupid and old is never a good combo. Those guys get no passes. It's a wrap.

What men need to understand about women in general, is that we have needs too. One major difference between us is that our needs typically extend past the bedroom to include a bunch of pseudo-scary emotional stuff which makes men uncomfortable. However, for the cougar, they do not extend past the sex. Cougars are focused and driven on physical pleasures only. We have no needs outside of the bedroom that don't focus on accessibility and getting back into the bedroom!

This desire and intent to keep the relationship strictly sexual works perfectly with younger men in their prime because we both have the same goal - amazing, non-stop sexual escapades with little to no recovery time! Stamina is the only thing that gets me emotional! I get all flustered just thinking about it! A man who can keep up with me in the bedroom, has the necessary equipment to get the job done (we've already established size does matter), and is a quick learner... now that's a wonderful thing that has been known to move me to tears. That's about all the emotion a cougar is ever going to give you.

There is nothing wrong with being forthright about your intentions and clear about what you want in a relationship. As cougars, we have a responsibility to be honest regarding what a man will mean to us and what role he will play in our lives over the next few hours, days, weeks, months or years. Otherwise their young tender sensibilities will think it's true love in minutes. What's the fun of being a cougar if you have to choose just one?

No, I will never be your girlfriend. No, I will never marry you. HELL NO to babies. And no matter how well you've mastered my favorite tricks, you can never move in.

Parameters and expectations must be stated up front. The most important rule - it's all about me. What I want and when I want it. If you become my favorite but are never available to me, no matter how legitimate the reason, I will make a call to someone else. It's not personal, it's sexual.

This policy is generally what irritates age-appropriate and older men who feel cougars are some kind of sell-out for wanting a younger variety. *So what.* Who the hell cares what they think? Why should any woman care about that? I don't remember any great outpourings of concern when they were horny as hell and trying to screw the entire female population during their sexual prime starting at seventeen! They wanted us to understand that it 'wasn't their fault,' or 'they just couldn't help it,' or my personal favorite, 'no matter what you hear out there, you're my girl.' Is it my fault many of them pretty much fizzled out shortly after that? No. It's also not my fault I like having sex for longer than ten minutes and enjoy a partner who feels the need to 'strive' for his absolute best performance over and over and over again. One who wants nothing more than the approval and excitement of an experienced woman, I can't think of one reason why I shouldn't be the one to give it to him.

Not even one.

When this is all over, he will walk away with a sexual advantage over his counterparts based on actual skills and not the 'bang-bang' theory of yesteryear. The self confidence will be genuine and not based on the souped-up egos of their jealous forefathers... some of whom think the 'bang-bang' theory is still valid. Dumb asses.

It's just logical. If given the choice, who would choose a forty-five year old man who may have one good run in him before needing a six hour recovery period, over a twenty-three to twenty-nine year old sexual dynamo who looks good, feels good, and is eager to please all night long? Not. Ava. G.

I have no intentions of selling myself out to accept years of wasteful sex during my prime. Why should I adjust to what society and old men feel is more socially acceptable for me and my life? Why should anyone? I am a woman who enjoys being hit on by younger men and have no problem hitting back... often. Don't get mad because I'm interested and turned on by a man whose main priority is finding and hitting all of my pleasure points. My sexual prime and the needs that accompany it are no less valid than yours were twenty years ago. Is it my fault you already peaked? Get mad! Do something! It could be the best thing for both of us if you do.

Chapter 5
Bang, Bang, Bang, You Know You Came!

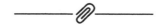

Dear Ava,

My dude is into aggressive and hostile sex all the time. He always has me twisted like a pretzel or stuck in wrestling holds. Sometimes there's just no way of getting out of his grip. I'm exhausted afterwards and in a fair amount of pain. I do not feel very involved in our sex and when we're in bed I'm pretty sure he hates me. Why is he so mad? I always tell him that he doesn't get extra points for hostility. Even though it's never boring, sex is supposed to be fun, right? I think this must be what prison sex is like.

Signed,
Tired of the Anger

Well Tired, I'm tired for you.

I'm no stranger to rough sex and aggressive behavior in the bedroom, but what you've described sounds almost criminal. This type of hostile sex doesn't sound like it would be good for anybody. It's no secret that men sometimes want to be rough. But it's not usually an everyday occurrence such as you've described. Sometimes an aggressive romp with fun dirty talk and appropriate tossing can be fun and add a nice dose of spice into your average run-of-the-mill sex life. But there are still limits and you should never be physically hurt from it as a result. For this to be his everyday normal mode of expressing his feelings for you is a bit much. There may be more to this than plain ol' simple carnal desire and sexual passion.

Your man reminds me of a gay friend who told me once that before he came out and accepted who he was as a gay man, he identified himself as being bisexual and had sex with women. He confessed that after a while he let that go because sex with women HAD to be rough or he wouldn't stay hard. It was his way of making sure he could 'make it through' and finish before his 'lower brain' disconnected and realized it was inside of a woman. I'm sorry to say, but this sounds like something your man might be struggling with.

Seems to me your man is fighting some internal demons and taking them out on you in the bedroom. Not cool. Men typically see women as gentle and refined. It's what makes us being a freak in the bedroom so exciting for them.

First, YOU need to be more aggressive about expressing your disdain for this method of sex. Sex is supposed to be fun. Sex IS fun! If you're not having any fun, then stop having sex with him! Sometimes a little pain after sex can be a turn on. But if you are in a "fair amount" of pain afterwards and feeling violated, it's time to speak up, expect results, or move on. I don't know anything about prison sex but that reference alone is enough to be a deterrent to getting naked for him again. Whatever happens just know that you and 'your girl' should not be paying the price for anything he's compensating for with his forceful disposition.

Think fun!

Ava

***

Rough sex is where it all begins for men and some never leave that trusted, rough space. Alone in their bedrooms they 'beat the meat' and brag about 'pounding out the pussy' with their friends. Because arrogance and cockiness rules the mind at an early age, they get all of their info from dirty magazines, television, and movies. Then it happens. A girl comes into the picture and all of a sudden, it's game time!

Once 'in,' a man knows how to do little else than bang and pump. And we make it real easy for them to think that's ok. We just lay there, legs spread and moaning like it feels sooooo amazing. It doesn't. But we are afraid to say anything, and don't even know what to say. He bangs his way through most of his twenties, and we master the art of faking it. It's a nasty and unfair cycle that happens and is happening, right now, in bedrooms all across the world.

This is where monsters are created. Men who feel they have the magic stick because every woman they touch explodes with orgasmic pleasures every time he touches her in any way. False. False. False.

But it's our fault. While they are pumping themselves into comas on top of us, we are looking at the ceiling moaning and groaning, all the while building up to that magical fake 'O.' We want our man to feel like he is putting it D-O-W-N... even before we know what that means. This feeling of accomplishment comes with a price. A hefty one. It costs us REAL orgasms!

Why? Because those early years of 100% orgasmic success with no effort whatsoever to *making* it happen, stays with a man! Shiiiiiiiiit. If somebody was in your ear for ten years or more, telling you how amazing you are with grunting moans of excitement and desire you would believe you were the bomb-diggity too! This pseudo sense of sexual confidence we create is consistent because all women do it!

Men never want to accept this truth: All women have faked orgasms... even with you! You will be hard pressed to find a man who believes that to be true or will even entertain the thought. And again...it's *our* fault. Because no matter if he's with you or the next ten girls after you, the sexual response he gets from every woman is always the same... "Oooh, Ahhhh. I'm about to cum. Oooh, Ahhhh. I just came. *That was amazing.*" Couples break up, and move on to other relationships, but the new women unwittingly continue the cycle. She goes through the motions just like we did. She has her fake O just like we did. And he rolls over feeling like 'the MAN' just like always. It's a vicious and nasty cycle which must be destroyed!

As women, we have to stop pretending sex is really great when it isn't! We have to demand more than a sexual fist pump and bang, bang, bang! We have to stop 'cumming on cue' and demand satisfaction! It does nothing but build a dangerous and false sense of machismo in every man. It declares the va-j as an orgasm-free zone for years and years and years... and years!

When a man, usually in his thirties, finally meets a woman who has stopped faking it, he gets MAD. How dare this frigid woman who can't cum complain about his performance, or lack thereof. How dare she act like he wasn't the absolute best she'd ever had, like every other women he'd encountered thus far. She wants the real deal O? Then why is she 'fighting it' and preventing it from happening? It would be laughable if the consequences weren't SO dire.

When a woman has finally found her voice and is able to communicate her sexual feelings to a man, it usually falls on deaf ears. Deaf ears we have created with lies and Oscar-worthy bedroom performances. Any woman in her thirties can vouch for this. While it's too late for many, most will eventually catch a clue. He will encounter a woman who not only tells him that pounding is not what works, but explains how he CAN get the job done, and then lead him down the correct path. I think most men will admit to seeing and feeling the difference between the faked orgasmic moments in their twenties, and the real deal toe curlers they genuinely cause in later years. The differences are staggering and impossible to miss.

I vividly remember the day my orgasm veil was lifted. I was twenty-three and in a relationship with my Navy man for close to a year. We were a hot couple. We couldn't get enough of each other, ever. We had what I thought was a lot of sex and I was mostly quiet through it all. He'd always ask me if I came, and I'd always say no... because I hadn't. But one night, when he seemed to be working particularly hard and asking me a lot, I decided to be vocal and give him what he so desperately wanted. I moaned. I pulled. I threw my head to the side and let out faint screams into his shoulder, and just as I'd seen in so many movies, I 'came' for him in a sexy-moaning-heavy-panting kind of way that told him, "Damn baby, you are the SHIT!" And so the monster was born. The rest of our sexual encounters were a wrap from there. I had to face to the reality that he would NEVER feel the need to even come close to 'working' that hard again. He didn't know what he had done to make it so amazing for me and he never would... because he didn't DO anything.

We did that show for another two years. I got better at it and he thought he did too. With no effort, no change in his actions, and no brief visits to the 'hood,' he became the sexual monster he'd been telling his friends he always knew he would be, before he ever touched a woman. Yes. I have contributed to the problem for sure. But NO MORE!

Let's face it, some men are never going to 'hear' the truth. Not from you and not from anyone. The first time I told a man I needed to cum he asked me why didn't I do it then? *Ummm... because that's your gig!?* He responded by saying it had to be me because this has NEVER been a problem with any woman before.

Noooo. Of course it wasn't babe, unless you count the fact that they were all faking it. He roared in anger and disbelief, "What did you say to me?!? WHAT DID YOU SAY TO ME?!" It's laughable now. But as the running theme in a man's psyche, it gets less and less funny as the man gets older.

While it's too late for many, woman can stop the cycle! It's our duty since it's our fault these men exist. Effective immediately, let's all vow to be a part of the solution and not a proponent for the 'bang-em-up-shoot-em' sexual problems of the past. Women should never fake orgasms. Never ever, for any reason. Spread the word. Tell every twenty year old woman on the street, and teenagers you think aren't having sex yet! Maybe if we can encourage these young women to want and demand more, they will get what they deserve, a real orgasm before they turn thirty-five!

Fellas, do your duty and always try to make it happen instead of thinking banging will get the job done. It won't! And no matter how hard you bang, or for how long, it just ain't what works!

For those of us in *cougarville*, we too have a responsibility... to teach the young ones how it's done. To show, guide, explain. This will not only enhance experiences with your guilty young pleasure, it will assure that his next age-appropriate girlfriend will be thanking you for those lessons all the way to the Oh-Oh-Oh Bank! *Trust Ava.*

Chapter 6
Boobies!

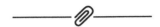

Dear Ava,

My boyfriend is addicted to strip clubs. Admittedly, I've known this for some time and it really never bothered me until recently. In an attempt to 'feed that need,' I went out and took pole and chair dancing classes. It was hard work! I have a whole new respect for those women. I've gotten really good at it and recently erected a pole in our bedroom and went to work. He loved it! The problem is, it hasn't mattered! He still prefers to go to the club and watch strangers, so now we fight about it! Now I feel disrespected and want him to stop spending so much money and time there. Is there anything else I can do to fill that void at home?

Signed,
Shiny & Tired

Shiny,   ✍

It's so hard for women to understand what all the hype is about since we don't 'get off' in this way, but it sounds like your man is like most others. As youngsters, boys get caught up in dirty magazines and porn. They can't believe they get to see a naked woman! As they get older, that doesn't change. This may sound crazy, but strip clubs feed the soul of the eleven year old boy who lives inside each and every one of them. It's the awe of seeing naked boobs, up close and personal, on REAL women!

Yes. Naked boobs! Men are simple and simple-minded. Now that they've seen and held a few boobs, the ones at home are no longer taboo and therefore less exciting. Just like everything else in their lives (cars, house, etc) they need to be able to compare and brag to their friends.

The excitement your man felt when he saw you doing dirty things on the pole was genuine. He will brag about it to his friends forever. But it doesn't kill the 'little boy' in him that wants to see new boobies. Everything men do is about the new. New boobs, new ass, new pussy. It's what motivates everything they do in life for always. It NEVER goes away.

I feel you on all the money spent. But let's face it, strip clubs are a business. They are set up to separate men from their money. As long as he's respectful to you and taking care of his responsibilities, he's entitled to blow his money any way he sees fit.

Unless he starts to cross some obvious lines (like befriending strippers), leave him alone about the club. So long as he's coming home hard and ready, enjoy the side effects and the free time. I'm sure you can find something to do with your new found pole skills...

I'm just saying,

Ava

***

I wish every woman would make it a point to visit a strip club at least once before making a big fuss about it at home. If you've never been, please go. You need to experience, at least once, what it's *really* like at the club. Most are seedy little nasty joints with bad DJ's, watered down drinks, and *very* average women on stage.

It's not like in the movies. It's not this popping place with the most beautiful women in the world who have the hottest bods. Far from it. It's filled with desperate people on the stage and in the chairs. Women desperate to be financially sound and independent from judgment under the watchful eye of parents, boyfriends, pimps, etc., and full of men desperate to be noticed and have the attention of a woman. Even the most famous spots in Atlanta and Vegas leave a lot to be desired. With grimy mofo's with unscrupulous business ethics and wandering hands as owners of these establishments, most clubs are a true reflection of that. Women may be less likely to make a federal case of an occasional trip to tittie bars, with a more clear picture of the landscape once inside.

Strip clubs are the epitome of pathetic. A bunch of unattractive men sitting around drooling at women who are out of their league in any other atmosphere. Here, the women are coming up to them and that feels goooood. It's the only place on the planet where an impotent loser of a man can have any woman he wants begging for his attention. They love having women, ANY kind of woman, walking by them and looking back *as if.* All she sees is dollar signs, but for him, it's an opportunity he would never have if not for the cash in his pocket. It's a win win.

It's a stripper's job to make a man feel like he's only one in the world that matters. It feeds into the fantasy he's paying for: That she would be there *even if* he had no money! The better the lap dance, the bigger the fantasy in his mind that outside of the club he might actually have a chance at *dating* Ms. Candy. Fat chance! It's the longing desperation that stretches across his face as realizes his lap dance is coming to an end. Ms. Candy will not continue for free, that is his reality. It's in that moment he realizes he's *still* not special. He's a mark. His wallet is the real star in the chair. As long as it's full, he is an ever-so-friendly dead president. Once empty, not so much.

It's also one of the most logical decisions a man can make in his limited power to *be* logical. If he goes to a regular night club he is likely to spend about $100 anyway, talking to women who probably don't want him any more than Ms. Candy. At the strip club he's at least guaranteed some attention from a pretty girl *and* gets to see boobies, for the same $100! Who can argue with that financially genius decision?

Feeling insecure about strip clubs is a waste of time and energy. Women should not get themselves all bent out of shape over them. It's just not that serious. Men are visual. They need to *see* stuff. It doesn't matter how amazingly hot their own *stuff* might be at home. It doesn't count. They will still want to go and see the bodies of *other* naked women. Drawing the line and getting your panties in a bunch will do nothing but make it that much more important to go. Think *denied* eleven-year-old child and it may be a little easier to understand.

It's not about cheating. If a man is going to cheat, he doesn't need the atmosphere of a strip club to do it. Helllooooo? Sex can be had for free. Flipping out when he comes home drunk and covered in glitter isn't worth the energy. If he's able to perform, take that! If he's not, roll him over and get it in the A.M. We really shouldn't concern ourselves with much more than that.

If a man wants to spend all of his money on some chick who rubs her ass on him for a few minutes, good for her! I don't see that as being any different from women who spend hundreds on shoes and purses they don't *need*. A want is a want. We all have our vices. If faced with the choice of a banging new pair of shoes, or a banging young gun with banging guns, I choose the young gun! I have enough shoes! Dropping a bill or two on a hotel room for the night or weekend seems totally worth it to me (young guns may not be as financially sound as one would like... don't care), while to me, the same amount on shoes just seems stupid by comparison!

Strippers *do* come in the male variety. However, most women I know, myself included, don't get a whole lot out of male strip shows. It's a fun outing with the girls for special occasions, but nothing more. Being logical creatures, I just don't think we get the point of being able to look but not touch. Frustration doesn't get me excited at all. Women figure, what could be more depressing than seeing all this great D I am *never* going to have at home? There are more exciting ways to blow cash.

I love it when I hear about all the women who are putting themselves into the 'good girlfriend' category because they have asked to go along on a strip club outing. It's laughable. Men don't work like that. They are excited to know you are *willing* to go, but they do not want you there! It never feels like the selfless move you intend. It only feels like a creative and sexy way you've designed to 'keep an eye' on him while he's at the club. You going there is not a true visit. He's not going to act a straight fool with you there watching him 'pretending' it's fun. The bad girl message you are trying to send him is lost in the translation. He's really eleven, remember? Taking you along to avoid an argument later is like getting caught by his mother when he was looking at a dirty magazine under his bed with a flashlight. Dead boner. That's all you've done despite proclaiming yourself as provocative and erotic. You're a kill joy. Stay away from the strip club with your man.

Men will always love to see naked women. Whether it's us in the bedroom, or Ms. Candy on stage. In their mind, neither is free. Who cares?! Relax. Take a deep breath. Cash in on whatever mood he's in when he returns, and head out in the morning to get those shoes!

Chapter 7
Ditch the Alphabet!

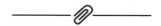

Dear Ava,

I just recently started having sex with someone new and it's been good. There is just one BIG problem, he will not go down on me. I figured it 'didn't work out' the first few times, so I finally asked and he confirmed he does not eat pussy. Of course he has NO problem with me slobbing him down and swears I'm the best at it! Am I throwing away a good man over something silly?

Signed,
Deal Breaker?

Ummm, yes girl, Deal Breaker!

I would have sympathy for a man who admittedly has issues with oral sex, but all of it... not just the giving part. If he recognizes it as a problem that he has a hang up about it then ok; let's see what can be done about it. But having issues with giving but not receiving is just plain selfish!

It's more than a deal breaker. His selfish nature runs deep and this will be the least of it. He will never put you or your needs first in any other area of your relationship either. Run, don't walk, to the nearest exit!

You may be in the majority of women who will never reach orgasm any other way. He sounds like one of those men who thinks he can just pound it out for about five minutes and be done. Sadly, too many women have accepted this in his past so he thinks he's 'doing the damn thing.' Be the first women to let him know, he's not! You will do him and the women after you a great service to stand your ground and simply keep it moving. I say take your superior 'slobbing' skills to someone who wants to appreciate you with proper reciprocation!

Quid Pro Quo,
Ava

***

Cunnilingus is more than what it's slang indicates as 'eating out.' It should more aptly be known as the *very* fine art of 'whispering sweet nothings' to your girl's va-j with your lips, mouth, and tongue fully engaged. It includes sucking and licking and kissing (no pecks please), the most valuable female sexual partner, the clitoris. So many men miss this and make the experience annoying and so much less enjoyable than it's supposed to be. Despite men *thinking* they have the gift of 'good tongue,' it is damn easy to f-up the whole experience by spending a whole lot of time circling the area (lips, etc.) and never landing on the runway (the clit) except by an occasional accidental passing. OH BROTHER!

First of all, let go of the alphabet theory of performance. There is nothing sexy about a pointy ass tongue jabbing at us while concentrating on some childhood version of the alphabet song in their head. We can tell, and it doesn't work. Men who gravitate to this theory of eating pussy suck at it. Think about it fellas, if it was easy you'd all be good at it, and trust, as a group... ya ain't!

You have to *learn* how to be good at it. You have to *want* to be *that* dude who can just shut it down. You can't just 'hear' about what to do and think it's going to kick in when you need it to. Giving good head is an art form and should be treated as such. You have to be able to follow your girl's lead to the *right* spots for her. It's not like riding a bike. You can't jump off of one and do the same thing on the next. We're all different even though some things are constant and can be winners every time. If you pay attention and are sincere in your efforts, you can become the standard by which all others are judged. Trust me, it's damn good leverage that will be useful later on.

Second, don't rush it. If you get down there and it's not already dripping wet, don't think your spit will do the trick. That's disgusting and fools no one. We *know* when we're wet. It accompanies being 'turned on.' If it's dry, you need to do *something* to get the internal juices flowing. Some of us don't need much coaxing and are wet when you walk through the door in anticipation of what's to come. But others need to be *motivated*. Passionate kissing usually works well... on the mouth, not the Va-j. Think high school first base type action. When you're rounding to third, check and see if *she's* happy but don't stick your fingers inside. For women, it's all about teasing, anticipation, and foreplay. Drag it out until she's practically begging for you to get down there, and then kiss your way to the final destination. Once you become a real expert at gauging your girl and her level of 'freak,' a quick taste off of your fingers for each of you should really get both of your engines revving.

When you arrive at the main attraction don't just kiss around it and jab at it. Spend a second or two breathing onto it before you reach in for a nice long warm kiss. A few things are of utmost importance - (1) Kiss the clit, not the lips; (2) Let go and give it some air. It's kind of like a fire and needs wind to 'spread'; (3) absolutely never engage your teeth in this area in any way. These lips cannot handle teeth! No biting! and (4) Do not hold it in your mouth while running your tongue over it furiously. It feels good for about three seconds and then the sensitivity of it begins to be uncomfortable and hurt. Just don't do it.

Third, know that it's not an easy gig. You may be down there for upwards of twenty minutes or more before you feel her legs start to shake indicating you're almost done. Instead of getting comfortable and easing up, grab that second wind and bring it home! Sometimes we may be able to squeak one by you without you knowing... so ask! If she says she's about to, or already did, *don't stop* until she physically reaches down and restrains you from continuing. There is 'this thing' called multiple orgasms. While elusive, it's possible *and* probable if you know what you're doing. Become good at this and be prepared to be in very high demand.

On the flip side, if after a few minutes, or thirty, you get the 'ol heave ho' from the area you probably suck at it and need some work. Depending on your age, you may get another chance. If she's able to give you instructions, follow them. Don't ignore what she's telling you works.

Even though practice makes perfect in other arenas, the truth is, you may not get many second chances with the same partner. If she tells you to stop, and gets dressed, you're done. If she grabs a condom and still let's you *in*, be glad and maybe try again later or pull out mid-stroke and go for it. Either way, don't act like it's *her* fault. Trust me. It's not. Women can and *do* cum. Just because it's not easy, doesn't mean it's impossible. Don't be an oral slacker.

Chapter 8
Silence Is Not Golden

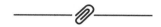

Dear Ava,

My girl and I dated in high school and were each other's first. We broke up junior year of college after six years. Ten years later we're back together but sex with her is completely different than I remember. She talks. She talks a lot. Dirty talk that's instructional. She's even mastered things she used to hate and refused before. Even though I'm having the best sex of my life I can't stop thinking about how she got so good at it, and I hate that. What can I do?

Signed,
Dirty First Love

Get over yourself DFL!

Are you serious?! You're upset because your ex had sex after you broke up and got good at it! Your ass is crazy! Old girl - true love - great sex! You hit the sexual jackpot and are too judgmental and stupid to appreciate it! You should be somewhere rejoicing over her improvements and happy she's willing to share them with you!

How dare you judge her for finding her sexual voice! Wonder no more about how she got so good - she was with a man who knew what the hell he was doing! They had a lot of amazing sex which was life changing for her! He relaxed her, made her feel comfortable enough to communicate her desires, and he FULFILLED them! You can stress imagining that picture or you can enjoy her skill set and be thankful she's not leaving it up to your stagnant ass to figure her body out because that gets old and tired real fast.

Surely you didn't expect to have your virginal girlfriend back at thirty something! Even though you lost your virginity to each other, she has grown sexually and you are living in the sexual past. You would prefer to have her laying there on her back as a receptacle like she did at seventeen? I'm almost afraid to ask what you have been doing over the last ten years. Hopefully, for your sake, you've graduated from the 'bang-bang' days of high school sex and learned a few tricks to please her! If you haven't you can relax because you wont have this problem for much longer.

I would suggest you get over yourself quickly and get with the program. If she's talking dirty you better learn how to talk back! If she's telling you what to do to make it better, you better be a quick damn study! And if she's making you cum like never before, you better figure out a way to reciprocate or she's going to get tired of your lazy ass and move the hell on... at least I would.

Don't you dare say a single word to her about this! You don't get to judge her and enjoy her. None of this is her problem. You should seek professional help to deal with this 'blockage' on your own. You boys are just never damn satisfied!

Grow up!

Ava

***

Listening to someone breathe on the other end of the line is frustrating, annoying, and dull. Lying ear to ear with someone, barely making any noises during sex except heavy breathing and an occasional grunt from an uncomfortable move or pressure is absolutely torturous. When we're young and have no idea what we're doing, this is all we know. Thankfully, we grow.

Talking about sex is important. Whether its purpose is to set out boundaries or discuss logistics, communication is key. If you are uneasy making sure you're both on the same page about the basics, like wearing condoms and how many you suspect you may need, how can you expect there to be any synergy once you are both naked and completely vulnerable?

Women are especially guilty of 'closed-mouth' syndrome. Fearful of what a man may think if we ask about or suggest condoms, we often put ourselves at risk unnecessarily. Learning to speak up can 'take the edge off' of tense situations. While I may not have always asked about condoms in advance, you can best believe the question was posed exactly when it needed to be. The timing of that proved poor on more than one occasion. Stopping a moving freight train is damn hard! It's also annoying as hell.

What man has a woman all worked up and ready to go and doesn't have a freakin' condom?! A dumb ass one! The idea that he may be willing to move forward without one can be a complete turnoff and a clear indication of his standard operating procedure of never using condoms with anyone. Women like to fool themselves into believing we are special. We're not. If he will run up inside of you bare back, he will run up inside of anyone else the same way. Don't be an idiot.

Carry your own condoms! There is nothing wrong with being prepared at all times. Having a condom in your purse is just responsible. Do it! Buy a box and always keep at least one on you. Even if you don't need it, you might have a girlfriend who does and she will certainly appreciate the gesture. (FYI - I do not condone women providing condoms on a regular. The one in my purse is for emergencies only. MY EMERGENCY. It doesn't mean he shouldn't concern himself because I already have one. It means if you don't have one, and I still want you after that idiotic and disappointing news, I will retrieve it. Otherwise, get off me. Game over.)

It takes *years* for most people to become comfortable talking during sex. Hell, it takes years for some people to feel comfortable talking *about* sex. But once you find your voice, it's almost impossible to silence. If you are someone who enjoys talking about sex, talking during sex is a natural and exciting progression. I personally have noticed a direct correlation between dirty talk and good sex. It's taken some time to get used to what comes out of some people's mouths, but even something borderline offensive is better than complete silence. Asking someone to take it down a notch is so much easier than expecting them to engage.

Waiting for someone to engage in the bedroom results in people tolerating bad sex for years, instead of speaking up. Once you get past that, and fall into the comfort zone of speech after the doors close behind you... it is so on! That nervous feeling of worry about what the other person will think quickly dissipates when the orgasms start to flow more freely. Once you figure out what to say, when to say it, and how it should be said, your sexual confidence skyrockets! But how does one *do* that you ask?

Finding your voice during sex depends. It depends on you, your partner, and your own personal comfort level with yourself. Being afraid to speak during sex will subside once you have some idea of what message you want to convey. Part of that can be acquired by getting to know yourself and coming to terms with what turns you on so you are in a better position to instruct and suggest. When you finally do have something to say, make sure it's something sexy *and* productive, even if it's non-verbal. Obviously moans always work wonders but most that are afraid to speak are not letting out any sexy moans either.

You can certainly 'speak' to each other without words. By taking a hand from one area and placing it on another, moving in a certain way, or moaning to indicate a 'job well done,' you can let each other know if something is good or working well. The message will be sent and received. But the verbal aspect can take it one step further. If you're nervous and scared about what to say or when to say it, start with short one or two word phrases. For example, once the hand is moved and placed where you want it, ask "Feel good?"

or offer words of encouragement like "Just like that," etc. "Damn baby" can usually spark some excitement but humans love nothing more than the sound of their own name. By replacing "baby" with his / her name (the RIGHT one of course), you can invoke remarkable physical reactions.

As we get more comfortable speaking, the sex gets better and better and often serves as foreplay to build up the anticipation of eventually being together. It leads to frank conversations before, during, and after sex. Phone sex and texting (photos and phrases) become second nature. Nothing we want to say is off limits. We can be as sexy, naughty, or raunchy as we want to be. Before we know it, we have less of a problem expressing what we want from sex, and more of a problem accepting whatever we're given. That's the irony of it all. We can go for years in silence, but once we start to speak freely and that door is opened, we will DARE someone to try and close it.

So often women are reluctant to participate in anything sexual that might destroy the image they may have of themselves, or the image of what others may have of them as being a 'good girl.' Having that pristine 'girlie' reputation is important to maintain for the world. But in the privacy of our bedrooms, our 'inner whore' can take over! We all have one and she is ready when we are. Be warned, she is crazy! Once her confident ass gets out, she is hard as hell to reel in!

Confident and crazy, she *knows* of the sex life you really want and she knows she is the only one who can be trusted to go get it. She helps you understand your body, your sexual responses, and how things work. She is the one who will find creative ways for you to please your man, and break down the wall that's kept you from experiencing euphoria in the past. Dirty talk becomes a natural 'conversation' and as her certainty increases, she can become impatient with slow learners, those who simply refuse to listen, and those without the proper equipment for maximum pleasure. She may have forgotten that men need positive feedback versus a list of 'all that's gone wrong.' She is not known for her patience, and the weak or selfish may not survive. Her ability to speak ensures she is done being a sexual repository and has instead opted for pleasure over compliance. Finding your sexual voice may qualify as one of your most vulnerable moments, but also one of the most sexually liberating.

Quiet sex is boring as hell and I've found nothing else to be an adequate substitute. Having found a young gun with a great body, great dick, and the oral skills of a sensei ninja capable of guaranteed and consistent multiple orgasms with indisputable assurance and surety (yea, he was THAT good), I was shocked to find myself bored senseless with the silent sex which followed. Silence is not my thing. Me talking to myself or getting no verbal cues or responses, is a waste of my time and a surprising blow to my well-deserved and hard-earned ego.

When asked about the eerie silence, he said he "just couldn't." Said he was "too involved in performing to talk." That it "felt too good" and he just couldn't speak... and that it "was weird." Weirder than dead silence?! I think not. I tried to hang in there for a while. I mean, he had other benefits that were UNPARALLELED (insert tear dropping here). I hated to see him go. But after a good year (he was REAL hard to let go LOL), I grew tired of restraining myself verbally, and he never really seemed to be ok with me being "short on time" right after his ninja moves were complete. Don't trip. I will call on him again. And he will cum...

Chapter 9
Not So Quick!

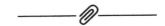

Dear Ava,

I am dating an amazing man who drives me wild sexually and the feeling is mutual. We have great sex and I really only have one complaint - we never seem to reach orgasm at the same time. Even worse, if he finishes first, I am typically left unsatisfied or topping myself off once he falls asleep or hits the shower. What can we do to make sure we climax at the same time?

Signed,
Seeking Simultaneous Satisfaction

SSS,

You use the word we a lot but it doesn't sound like your man sees this as a problem. As far as he's concerned you're having great sex. Period. If this is something you want to see change, you first have to make it known. Trust me. He is totally cool with you topping yourself off. In fact, he probably thinks that's what you should do since something is probably wrong with you (your inability to orgasm).

You have to remember, he's operating based on false knowledge from girlfriends past. As far as he's concerned he's been able to bang away and hear screams of ecstasy every time. You could very well be the first one who isn't willing to fake it for him. Good for you! You have your work cut out for you on this.

Regardless of where this all leads, you need to adopt rule number one right away - Me First. "If I don't cum, you don't cum... ever." Let's face it, once a man orgasms the whole session is typically over. There will be no efforts to please you after the fact. Just knowing you made him orgasm should be enough anyway, right? Pa-lease. You have to demand your orgasm first. If you allow things to progress before you reach the bell tower, shame on you. You can't get mad afterwards and have an attitude with anyone but yourself if you let that happen. If you don't cum first, you never will - accept that.

Talk to him to make sure he understands this as something you want. While he decides if he also wants the same, don't be ashamed to take matters into your own hands. You know exactly what to do to yourself and can while he's inside of you. This is NOT in lieu of rule number one. This would be your second orgasm for the session. Once he feels your walls convulsing around him, he'll be more inclined to experience that feeling every day.

Enjoy the journey!

Ava

Any scene portraying a couple moaning, groaning, and screaming in orgasmic relief together, just a few moments after ripping each other's clothes off, is a complete farce. Anyone who's ever had sex knows this is a physiological impossibility. No matter how turned on a person is, these things take time. Orgasms are just not that easy. Even when they flow freely, it's rare that both parties would be at the same place at the same time. The scene described above is a quickie and only he came. All she did was make the moment as enjoyable for him as possible by enhancing the experience with audible agreements and a warm body.

No doubt quickies can be exciting. Location, timing, frequency, and the opportunity presenting themselves, play into the sexiness of it all. For men, it's a win-win. They get in, they get off, they get to go back to whatever they were doing, completely satisfied. For women, not so much. No doubt we want that feeling of him being inside us more than anything. It's what makes sex so amazing. But for women getting in alone does not get us off and rarely results in an orgasm. That certainly doesn't mean we don't love it. Quickies for women are most often a preview of what's to come. It's an opportunity for us to say yes to making him happy, and grabbing a quick back-eye roll for ourselves. It only becomes a problem when every session is a quickie.

Quickies are not for everyday, unless there's some plan for an extended version later on the same night. Quickies are for couples. Couples who have lots of sex. Sex that is meant to satisfy both parties. If you are in a relationship, and all of your sessions are quickies, it's time for a conversation and an immediate change. While there is nothing sexier than grabbing five or ten minutes in a restaurant bathroom stall, it's less sexy to have that same type of session every night in your bedroom. It all goes back to rule #1 - Me First.

No matter how short lived a relationship may be, even a physical one, neither can afford to be afraid to speak their minds before, during, or after sex. Communication helps in reaching simultaneous orgasms. There is absolutely no way to achieve this lofty goal of mutual and mind blowing orgasms without talking and informing the other of what works, when it works, where it works, for how long it works, and what intensity is needed for it to work best.

When two people are willing to listen and learn from each other, it is possible to coordinate the three to five seconds it generally takes for a man to get an erection, with the varied longer time it can take a woman's faucet to kick in and start running. A common problem is a stalling in the conversation which requires a woman to take it one step further. We sometimes have to begin by explaining that most of what he has experienced to date has probably been a lie. Faking orgasms becomes an art form for us, and no man wants to believe it's ever happened to him. If you don't believe me, take a poll.

The average man will start by laughing. He'll find it amusing that you think any woman has ever faked an orgasm with him when you know what his touch can do. Try not to laugh out loud with him at the insanity of it all. Let him have his laugh. It will be short lived. Next, he will suggest the problem is not him or any of his ex's, but more likely a physical defect of yours. This will seem completely logical to him since you are likely the first woman to ever tell him such foolishness. Because of the extensive list of women who preceded you, he will find it inconceivable to believe all of them were lying and you are the only one who has ever told him the truth. If your relationship survives, he could begin to take a genuine interest in what your body is experiencing in future sessions. If not, your credit for providing him this valuable intel will hit him like a sack of bricks years later when a woman he wants to impress tells him the exact same thing. And then... a man will emerge in his bedroom.

Any woman who wants to effectively communicate with her man that his history of women having explosive orgasms at the mere banging of his genitals against hers, must first be able to express to him that it had nothing to do with him. It's a weird dynamic since he already doesn't believe you and thinks your fake orgasm claims are lies. He is replaying in his mind all those 'magical' moments from his past where he provided women the 'gift of himself' and they responded the only way they could... with dramatic and highly charged passion proclaiming uncontrollable combustion. It's a good thing female orgasms require no physical proof. None of us would have been able to manage this slapstick routine more than once or twice without detection.

Once you can convince your man it's not his fault, for the right reason, you will have a gold mine on your hands. A smart man will listen. He will learn to read your cues, stimulate your clit, and be inside you, at the same time. It sounds like a lot but trust me, it's SO worth the effort. When it happens, you will speak about it often, attempt to recreate it regularly, and rarely will the memory resurface without 'your girl' having her own tingling moment. I will say, attempting this feat with a young gun in his twenties could be futile. Greater success will be found with a man who has mastered dick control and can gage how close, or far, you are from reaching the finish line.

Being honest with a man about what you are experiencing can be tough. You don't want to say it, he doesn't want to hear it, and he will never want to accept it as truth. But with the understanding that (1) Quickies are for him, (2) Previous faked orgasms were not entirely about his 'bang-bang' method and depended greatly on his ex's sexual unawareness; and (3) Simultaneous orgasms are generally reserved for people who know each other's bodies very well and can be verbal during sex.

Once successful, be warned. This could make it hard to walk away from even the most unacceptable behavior later on. Being whipped by the dick is not cute.

Chapter 10
Is More Mo Betta?

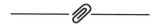

Dear Ava,

My boyfriend has become obsessed with the idea of having a threesome. We have been in a monogamous relationship for three years and he wants to "try new things," and bring another woman into the mix. Should I be outraged at the suggestion or simply insist on another man rather than another woman? Are there any restrictions when you involve a third party?

Signed,
The More The Merrier?

Merrier,

Being part of a threesome really depends on one thing: Can you handle it? Girl-on-girl action is a BIG part of your man's fantasy. Yea, he wants that 'special' attention from two women, but for men it's all about watching us 'get it on' with another female, up close and personal. Their own private show. You should know by now, it's not about pleasing two women, since most care little about pleasing just one.

Threesomes are not meant to be experienced with someone you truly care about. Not your boyfriend or girlfriend, and never your husband or wife. They are best left OUT of loving relationships. If your boyfriend wants to 'try new things' why not encourage him to consider exploring 'things' that will bring you two closer together sexually, rather than possibly make the initial rip in tearing you apart.

It's best to experience threesomes with someone you may be having a strictly sexual relationship with, or an affair. Yes, an affair. This way no one gets mad about what the other person is doing with the guest. No one goes home crying because he / she seemed to enjoy the other person more than they enjoyed each other. This adventure is best reserved for two people who like and respect each other but are not in love, and are not looking to have anything more than fun.

No man would EVER suggest a threesome that involves someone he truly loves and cares about. The mere suggestion is a red flag, denoting the end of your relationship somewhere in the distance. If you consider and agree to a threesome, be prepared for the ripples it will create in your relationship on the back end.

Know thyself.

Ava

I LOVE the idea of a threesome. I mean, what could be better than one sexy, hot, naked man in a room with nothing on his mind but pleasing me? TWO of them!! But nothing is EVER that simple is it? For sure, that is not what a man means when he casually makes the inference that a threesome would be 'cool.' Never do they imagine the invited guest to be another man. A man is only thinking of himself and his own desires when he suggests his girl fulfill this common and basic fantasy.

Even so, shouldn't we at least consider it if it's something he wants? I'm all about pleasing a man so listening to any idea is a good way to stay open minded no matter how crazy it may seem. We should always want to know where his mind is going, and we can always say no. Admittedly, with threesomes, there are lots of issues which must be addressed. By answering a few not-so-simple questions, you can make an informed decision you can live with. Ultimately, the power to allow it to happen or not, is completely yours. Just be prepared for the possible fallout no matter which way you decide to go. Are you ok with him having sex with another woman? If not, just scratch it right there.

Wanting a threesome is important for some men. Don't take it personally, it's just another hole in the room they want to dive into. And by dive I'm talking in a 'bang, bang' kind of way. The fantasy hardly involves an inner desire to sexually satisfy two women. It's completely laughable to think a man could even come close to that anyway. But he wants to have his way with both of you for sure. If you think you can handle watching your man enter another woman's body, then this part of the checklist is not an issue for you. But if witnessing that act will leave you wondering if he loves you, or if he wants her more than he wants you, or anything close to that, you should probably hold off.

In a perfect scenario, you both want to see the other person pleased to the highest degree. If that means intercourse, blow jobs, anal or whatever, with the invited guest, then so be it. This is where real emotions make it tricky. People say they can deal with it but they can't. I mean who really wants to see their man enjoying another woman? If you can't handle that, say no with the understanding you had first right of refusal. What does that mean?

It means he could respect your stance and suppress his urges, or expect you to allow him to experience it with two other women. Yes, that's right. Just because you said 'no' doesn't mean his desires subside. It's just like anything else placed on the table in a relationship and could be a deal breaker. Relationships are about sacrifice and this is no different. Either you sacrifice your stance on participating, sacrifice your monogamy long enough for him to fulfill it, or sacrifice who you are and the way you look at yourself as a result of either choice. It all comes down to how important fidelity is to both of you in the long run. This whole event is about him banging and watching, banging and watching. This brings us to the next area of concern in the threesome checklist.

Is it ok if the woman touches you? This is a two-sided logical question which leads into the next consideration - your willingness to reciprocate and touch her back. If your response is 'I'm not gay, so no,' this is probably the end of the decision making process for you. Please note, you do not have to be gay to follow through.

Again, sacrifices are made in relationships every day, some larger than others. Saying yes to a threesome tells your man you want to be that woman who pleases him. But it also simultaneously says you are 'cool' with being touched and pleasured by a woman, and vice versa. If you can't see yourself being kissed by a woman, touching a woman, a woman eating you out, and you doing the same, say no.

Even though the whole event might last only a few hours, once the night is over and you have both come down off your sexual high, will you look at each other the same? Will you question his love for you or see yourself differently because you enjoy being touched by a woman? It is not uncommon for a man to 'go back' to that woman without you. That too goes both ways, as women often report to being 'turned out' as a result and suddenly are seeking out same sex experiences independent of their man.

Finally, would he be willing to return the favor and make the same sacrifices for you? Yes, you read that correctly. Is he willing to invite another man into your bedroom for your enjoyment as well? Better yet, would you want that? Don't just defensively say no. Think about it and be honest with yourself. It's actually a much smaller sacrifice in the big scheme of things because such an adventure really is all about you. Men will argue, "...that's some gay ass shit!" But it sure wasn't gay when they asked you to eat another woman out was it? Because "that's different." No sir. It really isn't.

Lucky for them, no woman wants to see her man touching another man. No woman. That's a line we would never expect a man to cross and if they do, we have no desire to watch. I have met plenty of men who have done threesomes with their boys and explain the 'naked man dilemma' as an unwritten rule that dicks and hands of the other man should never touch or meet. Since the whole purpose of this little gathering is all about me and pleasing me, sounds easy enough and totally fair, so I CONCUR! Once you've agreed about that, it's time for limits and conditions.

Ava G. only has one condition - me first! This is a condition whether we are alone or discussing a guest. I cum first because it's been my experience that if I don't, I may never! That means our threesome journey begins with me, you, and a yummy man-guest of MY choosing. And just like he does not want to be restricted from kissing and sexual intercourse with his female visitant, I too should not be judged as he watches me enjoy another man grab my hips, pull me towards him, and slide inside to the sound of my inviting moans of anticipation and pleasure. See how that works?

It has been my experience that even if you clear the first two hurdles of the Ava Threesome Checklist, this condition pretty much cancels out everything. I have yet to meet a man who is cool with the idea of watching another man have sex with his woman. Men are selfish and egotistical creatures who think they are entitled to such treatment, and assume no woman ever dreams of bigger, better, more interactive 'human toys' in the bedroom. The last thing any of them wants is the threat of having a bigger, more engaged dick in the room, much less inside their woman.

It's a catch twenty-two. If your man is willing and cool with watching another man enter you, it's unlikely he sees you for anything more than sexual compatibility. If you're single, he will never marry you. Men want to marry women who are ladies in public and freaks in the bedroom, but not whores (and only a whore would agree to such a thing, right?). Even though you may have said yes for him, and never with anyone else, it won't matter. He will never see you as marriage material and will question everything he ever knew about you, and everything you ever told him. The really ignorant ones might even suggest loaning you out to friends.

The condition exists for several reasons. One, the sentiment of being fair and equal in our pursuit to please one another should be mutual. Why should I compromise if he is unwilling? I am not attracted to women. I have no desire to kiss, lick, smell, touch, play with, or eat another woman. Wrapping my head around another woman touching me is hard enough. If I'm doing all of that for him, I think it's only fair he provide a great big showing of faith that he'd do the same (actually less), for me. Two, I will be mad as hell if after we fulfill his carnal desires of being with two women, he decides he "just can't see it" to fulfill mine. Those are fighting words!

Each of these questions and many more need to be answered thoroughly before moving on to scheduling a date. For example, what happens if he wants his guest to be your best girlfriend, or someone he works with? That will certainly change the dynamic of the encounter since it could tap into your emotions.

Because we all crave discretion in such matters, it's important to be with someone who you respect and would never go around telling your business. This is another reason I truly believe the best way to enjoy a threesome is in a strictly sexual coupling which enjoys an unattached and noncommittal relationship (such as with a cougar, or in an affair). Certainly a married person would never go running around sharing details. Since cougars typically seek to make an impression, we expect chatter. The security lies in knowing their circles will never collide.

Bottom line, having a threesome is a risky venture. Considering and ultimately deciding to 'go for it,' needs to be something you both want, having weighed all the options and potential consequences for fun.

Chapter 11
Attitude &
Enthusiasm

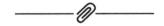

Dear Ava,

I have managed to have several boyfriends and never had to really argue about my disinterest in blow jobs, but not anymore. I'm 22. My current boyfriend is older and completely obsessed with the idea. I don't think I will be able to fend him off much longer. Not only do I think it's disgusting, I just don't get what's so great about it. Isn't it better to actually have sex than to try and simulate it with my mouth? It's not like a woman who can't cum without oral. Isn't creating an orgasm the whole point? Why are men so greedy? How can I get him to leave me alone about it?

Signed,
Ladies Don't

You need to get with the program Ms. Don't!

You're way too young, and way too old, to be carrying around this type of chip on your shoulder. This is

BASIC! While the women of the fifties were trained to believe it was an act of hookers and whores, it no longer carries that stigma. Woman finally got smart and realized it wasn't something a man was prepared to give up just because he married a 'nice girl.' Of course, those men weren't eating pussy either so who cares what they wanted.

The only reason your past boyfriends stopped harassing you is because they were getting it from someone else. Sex too! Don't kill yourself wondering if I'm right, I am. Your stance on how "disgusting" it is provides added incentive to keep your mouth away from it. That you hate it and don't see the point is advanced warning that you don't know what the hell you're doing.

You suggest sex instead as if the two were synonymous when any moron can see they aren't. Sex and fellatio are completely different. While the mouth and va-j have obvious similarities in terms of warmth and wetness, the tongue makes all the difference. If the va-j had a tongue, you might have a point. A good blow job is about attitude and enthusiasm supported by your lips, tongue, wetness, throat, and hands. Even the best developed va-j cannot compare to all of that.

Your attitude sucks! You have the nerve to call your man greedy when he is eating you to orgasm? You should want to please him and give him what he wants. Isn't that the point?!

If I were you I'd figure out a way to get over that BS and learn to love it. You are not only missing out on some sexy fun in the bedroom, you are conveying a message that his wants don't matter to you. If you don't want this man, dump him. If you do, please him.

It's that simple.

Ava

* * *

A man may never want to admit this, but blow jobs are nothing without emotion. Not the 'girlie' I-love-you type of emotion a woman may want it to be, but rather the intense, sexually aggressive emotion that results when a sexy woman wraps her pouted lips around his 'thinking head' and sucks. It feels really good. However, without the animalistic enthusiasm that a woman is going to die if she doesn't get it into her mouth RIGHT NOW, she might as well be sucking on his arm.

Men are simple, visual, egotistical creatures. Blow jobs don't have to be super creative or romantic. They just want to *see* everything so make sure you're comfortable being watched. It's all about the show for them, and knowing *they* are the reason you are behaving like a straight whore. It's *only* because of *his* raw irresistible machismo (wink wink). Attitude is everything and it has to be all about them and what they have done to *us*. Simple right? Yes!

The perfect and most memorable blow jobs involve an extremely horny woman who is visibly eager to make her man, or *this* man, feel like the only thing that matters in this moment is pleasing him in one of the naughtiest ways possible. Take the initiative! It starts the moment we lean in to his ear and ask his permission to suck it, and doesn't end until we've asked him where he wants to cum and thanked him for it.

The in-between time is spent making him feel as if the pleasure is all ours because we *need* this more than he wants it. How lucky we are that he is doing us this *favor* by *allowing* us to have him this way. Seventy percent of 'the job' is done before you've even unzipped his pants. We gain another ten assuming the right position for maximum enjoyment and his ultimate viewing pleasure. There are about as many fellatio positions as there are sexual ones but let's stick to a few variations of the most basic.

Face to face kissing against a door or wall is usually where you find yourself if he's just walked in. Hands wandering over the outside of his pants, take a long deep breathe when we feel that nice, hard hello against our hand. It warrants a deeper kiss. A moan. We should be tugging at his belt buckle like our life depends on it. Before we hear that jingling noise as the buckle gives way, we've talked about how much we missed it, how much we've needed it, and how we can't wait to feel it slide inside. And then we ask *permission* to say hello.

Before dropping to a sexy squat in front of him, grab a quick suck on the neck, and one or two more ravenous kisses. When you are face to face with his groin, tug on his boxers with your teeth before pulling them down to reveal the long awaited prize. With your hands holding onto the back of his legs for support, make sure the throat is nice and straight to minimize the gag reflex. There's nothing sexy about inducing vomit. Follow his manhood with your tongue until you can suck the head in and take it all in one, long, stroke. After a few minutes of sucking and swirling your tongue around the head, mouth closed, stand up for more kisses and push him into a chair.

Once he's in the chair make sure his ass is at the edge so *everything* is free because it's time to settle in between those legs and get 'comfortable.' Use of the hands and saliva are important parts of a great blow job. We can even make that sexy by looking into his eyes while licking our hand before placing it on top of the head and moving it down the shaft followed by a nice rounded mouth. Providing a wet and sloppy hand job will also help prevent his inevitable rush to go deeper as things get more intense for him.

Once your mouth is breathing hot air onto the head, and lips close around it - GAME ON for at least twenty minutes. Sucking the entire shaft into the mouth, be sure to tilt your head to the side a little so he can see and watch himself disappear into your mouth and feel the warmth of it at the same time. If you plan to have sex afterwards, you can have crazy fun with him until he just can't take it anymore. If this is in lieu of sex, every lick and every stroke needs to be productive or lockjaw is a real possibility.

Making sure the ass is properly exposed and poking out (imagine someone back there taking care of you the same way - and wouldn't *that* be nice), we can tease, lick, suck, and stroke making sure to apply most of the pressure on the underside, close to the head where all the nerve endings meet. Since the mouth serves as a preview of what the va-j has to offer, he'll want to place his hand on top of your head to 'guide.' News flash fellas - that's generally a no-no.

I haven't come across a woman yet who likes that shit. We tolerate it when we're young because we don't know how to make you stop. But as we get older and know what we're doing, it's just irritating and counterproductive. Either you trust us to do this or you don't. Want it faster? Speak. Want it slower? Speak.

Whatever you want, SAY it. This is not the time for nonverbal cues by thrashing yourself into our mouths and then wondering why our teeth are scraping the sides. This shit is not easy! It's called a job for a reason!

Contrary to popular belief the throat cannot be relaxed during fellatio and neither can we! In order for us to work our tongue, neck, and throat muscles in synchronization to take you deeper, we can't have you trying to kill us by ramming in! Death by dick would be hard to explain. Let us pull you in with our tongue as deep as we can *when* we can and it will be better for us and *amazing* for you. Unless you are playing in our hair, rubbing and squeezing our shoulders, caressing our back, or grabbing our ass...don't touch.

Looking up and maintaining as much eye contact as possible, increase the speed and veracity by breathing deeply and taking him deeper and deeper with accompanying moans. Be careful not to go too fast, too quickly. Keep the sucking and licking constant but controlled or your teeth will become an issue. We won't get into deep throating here, since it's so advanced. Just know by controlling the throat muscles it will allow him to *pass* the 'gag' area into your throat as if you've swallowed the head. Master this and you will *own* him. Trust me.

Staying rhythmic and synchronized helps get the job done. It gets tiring after a while so take quick breathers to realign your jaw and relax the mouth a bit by licking and stroking. For an extra long and well appreciated pause, push his dick against his stomach and run your tongue along the base and across his balls a few times eventually holding them in your mouth and swishing your tongue around them. Be *very* careful. No biting, tugging, or pulling. This will take your performance to a new level. Once you've gotten your second wind, take a deep breath, add in an emphatic "Mmmmmm," and lick your way back to the main attraction.

Lots of men will tell you they have never cum from a blow job. That was before. Never make any guarantees. But unless you are simply prepping for entry, this should be your goal every time. It takes time and is not easy. Also, because it may be a new feeling for him he may try to fight it and keep it from happening (it's the ego, remember?). Tell him not to do that. It's damn frustrating and will end with two deflated egos.

When he tells you he's close to cumming, this is the time to push your turbo button. Pull down and hold the base while sucking him in tandem to mimic what it would feel like if he were inside of you right now. When he finally tells you he's there, DON'T STOP.

Let it go everywhere. Either suck out every drop until you feel his body relax and collapse, or give him the fantasy of watching it squirt all over your mouth, face, neck, and boobs. (FYI - this is a great way to avoid having any in your mouth). Whichever works best for you, always let him watch, never try to kiss him right after, and be sure to follow it up with a sincere and sexy, "Thanks Baby."

If done properly, this can solidify your part in his pants forever. His pants, not his heart. Remember, this a man we're talking about. Let's not get crazy.

Chapter 12
Don't Play Yourself

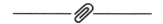

Dear Ava,

When I complained about my girl being too reserved in the bedroom, somebody told me to buy some toys to spice things up. I spent almost $300 and slowly brought things to the table. At first she didn't want me using them on her, but they changed everything. I'm pretty sure she doesn't even want to have sex with me anymore. She now has over twenty-five vibrators and toys and spent close to $1000! I can't remember the last time I was inside of her without a gadget before or after. She's way freakier, but I am being left out of the fun! What can I do to get her to focus on me and forget about all the electronics?

Signed,
Batteries Not Included

Blue **Print**

Well Batteries, you've made a common mistake.   ✍

You gave your girl a 'man' that requires nothing more than a flip-o-the-switch. I'm not sure there's anything you can do to reverse the effects of guaranteed orgasms. Guaranteed Orgasms?!! That's a hard act to follow.

It's been my experience that even women who absolutely love toys do not pass up on the real thing. Vibrators and such are typically a compliment to sex, not a replacement. They can be good in a man's absence but if she's insisting on their use regularly during all of your live sessions, you may have a bigger problem.

Your girl's 'reservations' in the bedroom might have more to do with you than with her. Maybe she was trying not to hurt your feelings by admitting she wasn't being satisfied. And maybe the fact that you thought to bring toys, and other more suitable sized penises into the room, was a sign to her that ya'll were on the same page. Now that she's hooked, you probably only have a few options.

The obvious and most favorable is to get better at giving her mind blowing orgasms on your own. Second, see if she will consider incorporating the toys less and less until you are the only toy left in the room. Third, see if she will agree to use them only on 'special occasions' or certain days of the week. Finally, keep her batteries fresh and be happy she lets you be there AT ALL. Honestly, if she is loving the toys that much, she really has little use for you. Be happy you are still in the room, or get a new girl and never consider toys again.

Good Luck!
Ava

***

Dildos, vibrators, and butt plugs - oh my! Nobody ever said this would be easy. With all the many 'fake dick' options available to women these days, it's a wonder men ever get a chance to make contact, right? False! There is no toy that can simulate the real thing. If a woman tells you she's cool with toys exclusively, she is mad as hell and refuses to admit there's no man worth letting in at the moment. A woman in her forties sitting alone in her bedroom surrounded by a bunch of toys is as lonely as if the toys were cats.

Toys are meant for fun and good times but some women take that shit real seriously. There are $100+ vibrators and dildos which light up, twist, are filled with rotating beads. It's crazy. Isn't the whole point to *replicate* sex and the real deal? I think I've had my fair share of sexual encounters, and I have yet to come across a man with a dick filled with pearls that rotates in two directions on ten different speeds. That actually *would* be fun! I'm kind of tired just thinking about it.

My first joint introduction into toys was three years after having my oldest child. Following six months of me refusing sex because "I wasn't ready to give that much of myself to anyone yet," my boyfriend took the liberty of enticing me with a big black, thick-veined dildo to speed things up. It didn't. We fooled around as always, and I let him do me with the dildo, but I really didn't enjoy it.

First, it had a weird smell like industrial plastic. It wasn't sexy. Second, his theory on how to use it was much like that of any real man in his twenties, 'bang, bang, bang.' Newsflash fellas: Few, if ANY women EVER come from intercourse. Take a poll if you don't believe me. Having that dildo inside of me didn't make me want sex any more or any less than I had before. Third, he didn't feel the need to *do* anything else since this plastic stick was inside of me. I never came (of course), and the session ended with me saying stop. What the hell is the purpose of these things again? I had no idea and evidently he didn't know either. I washed it, dried it and threw it into a draw, never to be used again.

Fast forward to two months later when I finally gave in to him. It was a long awaited moment for both of us. Passions were running high and we could barely keep our hands off each other. When he finally slid inside it was like he hit a bell and I instantly missed the dildo. I think he must've missed it too because he was stroking me like he was ten feet long and damn near falling out every time. You are NOT the dildo my friend. How can your depth ratio be *that* off at thirty-two?! Uggghhh! You can't be daddy long stroke with five-six inches. I'm just saying.

I felt nothing but disgust at that moment. I'd waited eight months for NOTHING. I found myself wishing I'd slept with him the first night and saved myself the build up to this fruitless moment. Later that night I went searching for the long lost dildo and couldn't remember what the hell I'd done with it. We broke up less than a week later. Six days longer than it should have taken. Learn this lesson fellas: Never buy your girl a toy that's bigger than you. I don't care how big or small you are, let this be a rule you live by.

The dildo eventually resurfaced and tormented me a bit more. I washed it again trying to get rid of that industrial smell (which refused to leave), and left it to dry against my shower door. Later that evening I was horrified when I realized my teenage nieces had been in and out of that bathroom all day during an earlier visit. I was so embarrassed! In disgust and shame I threw it into a huge box I'd been tossing papers and crap into for trash pickup and drug it to the curb. That night it rained and when the trash collectors picked up the box, the bottom fell out. When I saw all the trash in front of my house, I went to get a trash bag and collect as much as I could so I could still throw it into the back of the truck. When I returned, they were tossing around the dildo and waving it at each other. I ducked back into my house and made it a point to never be around on trash day ever again.

I'm sure most women have had at least one vibrating toy. I think the most common is the bullet. I've actually seem them in the ninety-nine cents store and received several as parting gifts at lingerie and bachelorette parties. It's a powerful little beast and if you're not careful it will have you 'jumping' in less than five seconds. I have a girlfriend who keeps one in her glove compartment and uses it almost daily while sitting in traffic after work. That's one way to pass the time.

I've been known to pull out a bullet or two and handle things myself. It can for sure become addictive. It's an efficient little invention. However, I've found after excessive use it can desensitize the area to the real thing. Let's face it, tongues and dicks don't buzz or vibrate. As a result, when with an actual man it takes longer and requires more to 'finish' and that's no fun. I tossed my bullets years ago and decided to use what every man has in his arsenal, fingers. It's a much more natural feeling that *can* be replicated during a live session, it's quiet, and I think it's even helped me to know what works for me. Toys just piss me off now. A reminder that I am alone and doing this myself! I don't think anything can top off an orgasm better than the feeling of *him* sliding inside afterwards. *Real tears*

I'm pretty sure I've gotten all I can out of any toy situation and learned some valuable lessons in the process. (1) Don't hold off on sex for too long. If it's bad, you can get out and you've wasted little time. If it's great, GREAT! (2) Bad sex kills all emotion as easily as a flipping a light switch. (3) Bang-bang sex doesn't work with a man, or a toy. *THAT'S* why they make em' do all those light saber type tricks and vibrate! Never let your toys surpass your man. If that happens...it's time for a new man!

Chapter 13
Open The Back Door

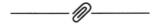

Dear Ava,

I am not gay and do not think about having sex with men, but lately I have been dying to try anal sex (giving, not receiving). I've heard mixed reviews. My girl says she is terrified and not a whore. Is this something that most women are against or secretly want to do? What are the general 'rules of engagement' on initiating? I am intrigued as a friend described his girls' orgasm as mind blowing, and I want to have that effect on my girl as well. How can I convince her to let me in the backdoor?

Signed,
I Want In!

I Want In,

You are not alone. I definitely think most guys want it. Some will admit it and those who don't are probably afraid of being called a homosexual if they do. Women generally see it as a prize and we don't run around handing out prizes to everybody.

It all boils down to trust. Talk to her about it. Find an article where a woman describes it as an experience other than painful and share the info. Be smart and don't embarrass or pressure her about it. Definitely do some research. At least one of you needs to know what to do and HOW to do it. You will need to be patient with her for sure.

Anal sex takes time. You can't just slide into the backdoor. No matter how wet you get her for vaginal penetration, she will NEVER create enough lubricant for anal entry to be enjoyable. You must invest in a good lubricant and use plenty of it.

Remember, it's COMPLETELY her choice. She sets all the rules for her body and what you can do to it. I firmly believe this decision needs to be made on a case by case, (or dick by dick) basis. It's one of the 'oh so rare' instances where smaller is probably better.

She decides!

Ava

***

The thought of someone entering an area designed for exits only can be terrifying to a woman. It takes our thought process to the most logical place - the bathroom toilet. As much as we may not want to discuss or admit it, we've all had unpleasant moments in the restroom where constipation turns an everyday natural human body function into what feels like 'giving birth' from the wrong canal. THAT shit hurts like hell (literally). The thought of allowing something twice that size to *enter* is almost inconceivable. Despite the intrigue of trying something new and expanding our sexual horizons, anal sex starts out as a big 'eewwwww!'

Anal sex is also very one-sided. Is it absolutely hilarious that men are quick to make the suggestion, or 'accidentally' poke us in the ass in the heat of the moment, but if we even get close to their nether regions with so much as a wadded up bed sheet then all of a sudden they are standing upright, butt cheeks tightly clenched, using the deepest voice they can muster saying, "Noooooo!" Is there really that much of a difference? I mean, asses are anatomically the same and serve the same purpose on men and women. It's really not a portal *meant* for entry for either of us. Throw a blindfold on and it's doubtful anyone would know if that ass was attached to a man or a woman. I'm just saying...

Anal sex is a tough one (no pun intended). As much as I would like to say I'm a member of the club, I have always been super chicken. Why? Cause that ish is gonna huuuuurrrttt! I've agreed to it and changed my mind every time. Too scary. I'm not into *that* much pain in the bedroom. Aside from the obvious physical trepidations, I've heard too many firsthand horror stories to count. Ring O' Fire?!? *What?* Entry of a penis described as feeling like an internal flame is deterrent enough for me.

It seems only logical that one might be concerned about what's *in* there. How can having a man's dick covered in crap be sexy? But I was told this was never the case. It was a 'clean' area. Completely free of said packaging until just before you felt the 'need to go.' But this doesn't keep women from wanting to be sure.

In anticipation of allowing her man to clear the threshold of her forbidden backdoor, a friend of mine began prepping for the moment hours prior. All of the usual washing was accompanied by an enema. She wanted to be sure the area was completely free of anything 'unpleasant' so as not to further impose on her already vulnerable state of being. Feeling clean and fresh, she was all set to go.

After a full round of 'regular' sex, it was time. With all the required and recommended benzocaine and lidocaine numbing lubricants, he started to slowly rock inside her anus until the head of his penis was able to break through. She explained the initial discomfort as tolerable. About fifteen minutes of slow rocking and gentle thrusts forward, he was in. She explained it as "painful pleasure" equivalent to a sexy slap on the ass that stings and excites at the same time. But the feeling quickly vanished as she felt an enormous amount of pressure in the area. She ignored it for as long as she could before realizing what was happening... the enema was kicking in! Before she could push him out and scurry across the bed to the restroom, the sound of a bad spigot emanated the room and her man and the wall behind him was covered in crap! Good thing it all took place in a hotel room!

Horror stories aside, I have a girlfriend who not only loves it, but prefers it. She professes the area is tighter, orgasms are more intense, and the risk of pregnancy is nonexistent. She and her husband swear by it and recommend it whenever the conversation or opportunity presents itself.

As self-professed experts they don't recommend rushing into it. They suggest taking baby steps to 'prep' the area and gage the feeling before taking that final step by inserting fingers, toys, and any other 'objects' that will loosen the walls a bit and offer enjoyment to her. A good time to throw it into the mix is during oral. Since a woman is relaxed and enjoying the moment, she may be pleasantly surprised by the insertion of a finger moving rhythmically in step with all the other good things happening. Over time, another finger and another can lead up to the big moment and cause it to be relatively painless and enjoyable overall.

If you decide to break your backdoor cherry, and it's a first for both of you, be sure to have all the lubricant and time you will need to experience maximum pleasure. And do share the details with your girl Ava. I will need a bit more convincing to let the big d**ks I crave, in through the back door. Of course, I do WANT that crazy intense orgasm so please... convince me.

Chapter 14
It's SO Not Personal

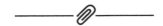

Dear Ava, ✍

I've been dating my boyfriend for almost 15 years. We've never lived together, (because I've refused) nor do we have any kids together. Neither of us has ever been married but he knows I've always wanted a family. Two years ago, he fathered two children by two different women in the same year, and I left him. I'm ashamed to admit, it was a temporary departure. I forgave him and eighteen months later we reunited. However, he has spent the last three years accusing me of cheating on him and says he can't trust me. Ava, I have never done anything but support and love this man. What's going on and should I even care to find out?

Signed,
46, Confused, and Childless

46CC,   ✍

You already know the answer to your question. Your man has failed miserably at loving you, and he's irritated that now you both know it.

I'll bet it never occurred to you while he was begging for you to take him back that he would eventually flip-the-script and blame everything on you, did it? Well, that's exactly what he's done. Don't feel bad. It's what men do. At the end of the day, you forgave him for everything and took him back. By doing so you promised to love him as if nothing ever happened, and give him your heart again. And you have lived up to your end of the deal. So why all the drama when he is the one who disrespected YOU by laying down with those other women without protection? It's simple: Your man's internal guilt will forever make you guilty.

Here's how it works: He remembers all of the logical things you said to him when you left, and in his mind, you could never forgive him, nor should you have. Even though your actions were sincere, his guilty mind refuses to allow him to take your forgiveness seriously. It's because he knows with absolute certainty that if the situation were reversed, he would walk away from you and your f'n baby and forever be done.

Basically, he has convinced himself you are back in his life for other more sinister reasons, like payback and revenge. So instead of accepting his failures and your forgiveness, he is more concerned about making sure you never have the opportunity to hurt him in the same way he hurt you. He just cannot wrap his head around why you would ever love or forgive him after all that's happened. He's afraid to trust you with his heart because of the way he betrayed your trust when he mishandled yours. He will never believe otherwise, and he really doesn't deserve to. You've wasted enough time with his ass. Leave him with his baby-momas!

Get your life back,

Ava

***

I have often wondered what makes a person go back to an ugly relationship or situation. When a person cheats or conceives a child outside of a marriage or otherwise committed relationship, what can be said to convince the injured party to stay? Isn't it fair to say if someone cheats there was never love to begin with? In my youth, I would have said yes. A man or woman who cheats does so because they do not have any love for the person waiting at home. Experience and life have caused me to disagree.

Relationship gurus and those qualifying as sex experts almost unanimously agree that when people cheat it's not truly physical. They claim there's an emotional pull in the relationship and people cheat for companionship and conversation. I'm sorry, that's just plain bullshit. People surely cheat for different reasons, and there are some women who feel an emotional pull in everything. But men? When has a man ever been moved by anything more than what 'emotionally pulls' them from below the waist? Sound mean? Don't care. It's the truth.

When a man cheats it's RARELY, if ever, emotional. I have found that men cheat for four main reasons: (1) Because they *want to*, (2) Because they *can,* (3) Because the *opportunity* has presented itself, and (4) Because there is a *willing participant*. Basically men cheat for no reason at all! Notice how none of that has anything to do with whomever may be at home- girlfriend, pregnant wife, mother of his kids, or high school sweetheart and wife for the past 25 years. All that matters is what they want, if they can get it, when it can happen, and with whom. That's it.

If there's anything I wish I could stress to women, it's this: His cheating has NOTHING to do with you. Nothing at all. EVER. He didn't cheat because you aren't making him happy at home. He didn't cheat because you said or did anything. He didn't cheat because he doesn't love you. He cheated because HE COULD! That's it. No big psychological guesswork. As women we take things so personally and it's so not personal. It is just not that deep. How could it be when MEN themselves are not that deep? He cheated *because he could.*

That's not to say it's ok or I agree with the logic. It's just an offer of understanding in the thought process. I do not concur with the theory of it being in a man's nature to cheat like many will profess. That's also bullshit. Monogamy is no more a natural state for women than it is for men. Men are no less capable than women of being monogamous. It's just that not very many women see the point of it. I see the problem as one more of semantics versus emotion.

One could argue that no one is too busy to cheat. But I think sometimes, women are. Not so much physically busy, in the sense we have a lot of running around and things to do, but mentally busy as in, 'no time to deal with *another* man's bullshit.' It's the same logic that prevents logical women from wanting to deal with married men.

Let's face it, sometimes a married man is the perfect candidate for a sexual partner. When a woman is in an 'in-between' place of ending one relationship but not really ready to be bothered with another, a married man would slip in line perfectly. First, they aren't looking for anything more than a good time. Second, their time is not their own. That means we don't ever have to worry about him getting mad because we didn't call for a few days. His popping up in places he doesn't belong is slim to none. And if we don't want to be bothered we can just ignore the call or text with no real repercussions. As forbidden sex it would be GREAT, and when you're done, you're done. No drama. No hassle. No big deal, right? WRONG.

Wrong, wrong, wrong! Because men have no idea how to handle any of that without getting their spouses suspicious or outright getting caught! It's what keeps married men safe from me personally even though they'd fit perfectly into my noncommittal roster. The last thing I need is someone's wife or long time girlfriend coming after me thinking I want her damn man. I don't. Sadly, men cannot be trusted to protect the relationship at home so I just prefer to not take those types of chances.

If only they were better at this game they think they have mastered. So many women and hearts could be saved if men could just 'up their game' and be better at chasing and following through on all that ass they feel the need for. Why is it a man can never seem to cover his tracks? Damn! This pisses women off more than the act of cheating. Have the decency and common sense to not get caught! (1) USE CONDOMS, (2) Don't go running up inside of anyone we know or who might know us, and (3) Don't tell stupid lies! There's a respect level which must be met.

That means you should never put us at risk for disease or make babies. We should never get a call from some random chick for ANY reason. And for goodness sake, let the people who you include in your lies KNOW they've been included! This is just blatant stupidity if you don't. The inability to adhere to these four basic concepts is what costs people their relationships, and rightfully so. You should also know that unless you have been raising a child you didn't know wasn't yours, received a phone call from some random man professing his love for your girl, or caught your wife in several stupid ass unbelievable lies, a woman you care about has likely extended to you these very same courtesies.

Because we *are* good at handling our business and keeping it moving, men have thoroughly convinced themselves that women don't cheat; not on *them* anyway. It's kind of funny really. No matter what kind of low down dirty crap they are slinging around on a daily, they still never think for a moment we might be silent to it because it leaves room for us to do the same. I mean, why make a stink about something that clears up my time and availability as well? PA-LEASE. A man who wants to party all the time, hang out with his boys, and be 'out there' living the pseudo-single life should always assume his girl is doing the same thing.

Even if she's not, she *should* be. What's good for the goose mofo...

And yes, a woman may entertain a man who feeds her emotionally if the one who's supposed to be there isn't doing it. But it's not a prerequisite so long as (1) We *want to*, (2) We *can,* (3) The *opportunity* has presented itself, and (4) There is a *willing participant.* Oh, and there is ALWAYS a willing participant. KNOW this.

Cheating involves risk. It's even more risky if you're bad at it. If you are cheating and taking crazy chances at getting caught, you don't *deserve* your family and whatever you've got waiting for you at home. The best thing a cheater can do is respect their spouse enough to protect him / her from the drama of carelessness. Those who can, will lead happier lives at home. Those who can't, may suffer the consequences of meeting the 'Bobbit' which exists in every woman.

Don't ever say you haven't been warned.

Chapter 15
Listen Up!

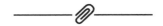

Dear Ava,

I always manage to find myself in embarrassing situations in the bedroom. If it's not a huge pimple on my ass, it's the irresistible urge to fart. There's always something that keeps me from feeling 100% confident about the pending joy. It's so unfair! No matter what I do to make things awesome, I'm always waiting for that embarrassing moment to hit. It's like I'm jinxed in the bedroom. I wonder if it's like that for everyone, or if I should just stick to doing things myself. Suggestions?

Signed,
Unlucky 13

I can't help but laugh 13.

Everyone goes through moments like these. EVERYONE. No matter how well orchestrated, every moment in the bedroom cannot be planned or anticipated. Things are bound to go wrong at some point. It's human nature.

It may seem like you are experiencing more than your fair share, but you probably aren't.

It can be worse if it's your first time together. The last impression anyone wants to leave on a newbie is a bad one. But some things are just unavoidable. Heads bump, va-j's 'fart,' and people lose their balance and fall off of beds. Believe it or not, most of these mortifying moments can be lessened by laughing at yourself and the situation. So long as there's no serious injuries that end in a trip to the ER, you can laugh it off, and your partner should end up laughing with you.

If they overreact, get all offended and act crazy about it, they probably don't deserve to have you anyway. Shit happens. These random mishaps should really take the pressure off of both parties to be perfect, and actually lead to some pretty amazing sex.

Believe it or not, you can and will recover from embarrassing situations. Take it from someone who has had, and caused, a bloody lip or two simply by trying to change positions too quickly. A few quick giggles, a slap on the ass, and all is forgiven and the great sex continues. Bottom line, we can't always be the bedroom goddess we imagine ourselves to be, and neither can he be that god. Learn to laugh at yourself and each other, and these moments will become less of an issue for either of you.

Have fun!

Ava

No one ever said sex would be easy. Sex is generally not 'easy,' but it should always be FUN! If you're not having fun with your partner, just stop. There *is* fun to be had! It's kind of like rides at an amusement park. You walk around the park for a while and pick one you think will be awesome. You wait around and stand in line, but when you finally get on it makes you sick or dizzy. You may even feel like you wasted your tickets and should have used them for the ride right 'next door.' Would you just keep standing in that same line? Just keep riding and getting sicker? NO!! It's the possibility of an exciting ride that remains the motivation to keep looking and standing in different, equally long lines. For every five decisions to take a bad ride, you may get one awesome ride that you want to go on over and over again! Eventually, it *will* payoff and the fun that follows is *entirely* worth it!

Once you find that great ride, keeping it fresh and exciting becomes vitally important. Each time you ride you get a little braver. You might open your eyes the second or third time around. Your tight grasp on the restraints with your nails digging in gets looser. Eventually you come to trust the ride and know what to expect at certain peaks, twists, and turns. Before you know it, you're riding with no hands in the first car ready to experience all it has to offer with little to no fear!

Society teaches us that new is better. With sex and sexual partners, we seek to prevent feeling the need to seek the new, and instead look for ways to 'newly invigorate.' What often results, is toys, experiments, kinkiness and fantasies lived out in bedrooms around the world. With all of that comes additional risk. Risk of being vulnerable, risk of embarrassment, and even risk of injury when things don't go quite as planned.

It shouldn't really matter so long as you are laughing about the various mishaps *with* each other versus *at* each other. If we are willing to cut ourselves some slack, things will be a lot less uncomfortable when a crazy cramp, kick in the face, or unexpected fart find its way into the bedroom. All things considered, there are specific no-no's which are much harder to recover from, are not funny, and are much less forgivable.

Imagine you are riding your man, legs interlocked behind you, when you decide to shift positions for better leverage. With both feet now planted firmly on each side of him, you continue bouncing inevitably hitting, twisting, or banging him into an inner 'wall.' You feel the weird bump, he feels a snap, and your sex life together is effectively over, his maybe forever. This is exactly what happened to John Doe and Mary Moe of Massachusetts in 2005 (I swear I didn't make that up). In this bizarre twist of events, John *sued* his long time partner for fracturing his penis because it culminated in the immediate need for emergency surgery and turned into a long and painful recovery period. In the end, the judge ruled Mary was not at fault since the two were having consensual sex and she had no intent to injure him. However, John suffered sexual dysfunction that has thus far been untreatable, which means they both lost.

Ironically, trips to the ER are not that uncommon. Couples can get stuck in all kinds of complicated positions, and va-j's can cramp up around a man during orgasm and squeeze so hard release is impossible without medical intervention. (FYI - muscle relaxers generally do the trick). These are extremes at the far end of the embarrassment scale. Much more common are the inadvertent mistakes and mishaps which occur to almost everyone at least once.

Screaming out the wrong name, or even whispering it, is a common and complete mood killer which is rarely overlooked. Depending on your relationship and timing, it could be a permanent deal breaker. Attempting to diffuse the anger with laughter might actually get you killed. A quick thinker might get creative and scream out other miscellaneous names to try and diffuse the situation. If it works… GOOD FOR YOU! If it doesn't, it's a lesson learned. (FYI - call every one "baby" and no one gets hurt.)

This is a good time to point out that listening is a good skill to master in the bedroom. A common complaint among women is the inability of a man to simply listen and follow instructions. There is nothing more frustrating than finally finding and being comfortable with your 'sexual voice,' only to have it ignored. If a woman says harder or faster, you don't get to increase both for two seconds and then go back to whatever it was you were doing. If you do, that elated moan you heard when you increased as asked, will be quickly followed by a much more frustrated sigh of annoyance when you stop.

Equally infuriating is the execution-style response to "I'm about to cum." That kills orgasms dead in their tracks. I have not figured out why any man would think this is the perfect time to do something *different.* It isn't! It means keep doing what you're doing and you'll be done! Anything less than that results in an angry woman and a tired man. Hint - the last thing to do when a woman proclaims this statement during oral, is hold her clit hostage in your mouth and suck on it or beat it furiously with the tip of your tongue! If you have learned nothing today, let this be it! It ruins everything *and* hurts like hell!

Also strict no-no's are adding lubes, jellies, and other crap to the mix without so much as a three-second warning. I have no idea what genius decided vapor rub would feel good on a clit, but it's a problem more than one woman I know has experienced. Stop that today! It burns like hell you idiot! Not to mention it's not edible! If you want to stop, STOP! Don't ruin me for less lazy henchmen in the days that follow! Speaking of lazy henchmen...

Nothing will send you running back to your ex like a bad experience with a newbie. There's something about *knowing* what you're going to get, versus hoping for the best, that makes this move somewhat inevitable. It totally sucks because going back doesn't mean you want 'all-in,' it just means you miss the sex! If you broke up because your ex is an ass, you end up feeling like you failed yourself on some level. Don't. It's human nature to go back to what's good. I liken it to visiting the same restaurant repeatedly and ordering the same meal no matter how much you intend to try something different. There's comfort in the knowing.

So if you cave and give in after ignoring countless emails, texts, and phone calls begging for just that, just go with it! I have found myself ruining the enjoyment of it all by laying there regretting the decision and having internal arguments with myself about being 'so much better' than this. I usually just want him to shut up and stop reminding me of *why* I said I would never go back. In pursuit of great and guaranteed sex, I have learned to shake that creepy feeling of disappointment and focus on the purpose he is serving for the moment. Whatever you ultimately decide to do about those weak moments, get over it quickly. There's no point in beating yourself up over something you thoroughly enjoyed. So long as you don't sign on for more than the physical, you should be straight.

In Conclusion ...

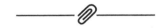

If you've learned nothing about me in the preceding chapters please know this:

I have learned a great deal about men over the past twenty years or so. Some lessons have been hard. All have completely changed my response to different situations. My previous attitudes and much of my behavior in the past was a complete waste of time.

With a thorough understanding of myself as a sexual being, I see things differently now. I take nothing a man does personally. I still get angry. But it has more to do with not getting my way than having my feelings hurt. I want what I want when I want it. Doesn't everyone? I've found that the quicker you are able to admit that to yourself, and to anyone who *has* what you want, the more often you will get it. I am living my life as a result of lessons learned and realities accepted. It works for me.

As a young adult, I spent much of my twenties and thirties looking forward to dealing with 'grown men' who had tired of the game playing and insensitive decision making that required they take no one's feelings into consideration but their own. Now in my forties, I realize that day never comes for a man. They have already become who they are going to be by the time they are thirty-five or younger. They just *have*.

Last year when my father's girlfriend of fourteen years called me frantically looking for him following several unanswered phone calls and a visit to his newly vacated apartment, I knew this *for certain* to be true - they don't change just because they are old. Since I had not spoken to him myself for several days, I called to make sure he was OK. When he answered and I explained the reason for my concern, he said they had broken up. I asked, "...does she *know* you've broken up?" His response? "She should know since I haven't responded to any of her calls, emails, or texts." Did you *tell* her you didn't want to see her anymore? "No. What for?" Ummm... seriously?! At seventy-six, my father proceeded to *move* into a new home and completely ignored her, *never* explaining why to anyone. He subsequently married someone else less than a year later. With men, it simply never ends.

Today, I recommend others to never ask me questions they don't want, or can't handle the answer to. I stopped lying to men years ago. Sometimes the truth hurts. Oh well. I don't have time for the alternative, which is a whole lot of game playing and extra effort I just don't feel like exerting to maintain a lie.

I don't assign or accept titles that define my relationships. As a result, I'm never cheating. Am I seeing other people? Hell yes. And that's my answer even if I only see that 'other person' once every few months. Relationships are a lot of work. I don't have time to explain to someone why I haven't called in a few days. The thought of wasting even ten minutes explaining that decision to any man is incomprehensible. I just can't.

Life can be complicated enough. I need things, *some* things, SEXUAL THINGS, to be easy. Young guns are easy *and* fun. So long as I continue to act responsibly with them, being honest with my intentions, it's perfect. A girlfriend recently asked, "Are you still seeing that twenty-something year old young guy with the eight pack abs?" Yes ma'am I AM! "How much longer are you going to be with these young guys?" For as long as I can girlfriend! For as long as I can!

Yours in freedom and inhibition,
Ava G. Black

About the Author

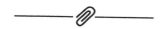

It seemed to take forever for Ava G. Black to realize she was navigating life with the wrong user manual, following the traditional female script for a sex life of light weight servitude, filled with humdrum canned and robotic 'Yes! Yes!' moments. She was bored and unfulfilled. SHE WANTED MORE! Once the decision was made to break free, everything in life was better and the exhilaration began.

Ava G. Black was your average woman moving through life in the most appropriate and politically correct ways possible. Careful to avoid imposing herself on anyone, or inconveniencing others in any way, Ava was a nice, likable woman who didn't make a fuss or stand out in the crowd. She was a good listener and friend, a loving mother, doting wife, and loyal employee. She enjoyed what most would consider 'a good life.' But as life often works out, the floor fell from beneath her, and before she knew it, she was a single mom 'maintaining,' expected to recover and get back into 'the dating world.'

It took some time, but she did just that. The process wasn't without major hiccups, but in the end, or the beginning, Ava found her voice and decided things would be different. No more pushing down what *she* wanted. No more settling for what people wanted to give her. And no more 'Yes! Yes!' moments that weren't genuine and hard earned! Ava began living her life *for her* and realized that despite all the hype and attention people give to sexual experiences, sex was actually *under-rated*!

For years she thought it was awesome and all it could be. Oh but how wrong she was! Going through the motions no more, Ava figured out key pieces to the male-female puzzle, resulting in better knowledge of self and a true understanding of answers to "Why?" … Why do women, why do men, and eventually... Why not!?

A Philadelphia native, readers have been enjoying her frank and candid insight into sex and relationships in Philadelphia's Urban Suburban Magazine for years. No stranger to radio and always ready to speak truth, Ava has advised women and men across the country on everything from the cruel reality of soul mates to 'reverse' threesomes, dick theory, and the power of the 'P.'

In Ava's first penned book, *Blue Print*, you will get to know her intimately and wonder why such simple and logical concepts have been so hard to grasp before now.

Ava lives gloriously happy in her 'new skin,' unafraid to admit to what excites her in the bedroom, and able to provide instructions when necessary! She suggests this book is perfect for any man or woman who wants the same!